Lyme Free Living

In An Infected World

Dr. Christopher Maloney, N.D.

ISBN-13: 978-1983784583

ISBN-10: 1983784583

DEDICATION

To all of us who live in Lyme lands. May we all find comfort and direction.

CONTENTS

ACKNOWLEDGMENTS

My greatest appreciation to the pioneers of ILADS, the hearty women and men who have bucked the system to relieve the suffering of Chronic Lyme. And my thanks to all the patients, the tireless foot soldiers of Chronic Lyme who have refused to be silenced by an apathetic system. You are my heroes.

Preface

It's time to stop the Lyme madness. We need to take a step back and really look at how we can live in a world where Lyme is continuing to spread.

Wherever you find yourself on the journey of Lyme, I want to help you live in that world. If you've just been diagnosed with Lyme, please read this book before you subject yourself to aggressive treatment. If you're a battle-scarred veteran of the Lyme Wars, I go into aspects of Lyme you may have missed. I also give you more treatment options.

If you or a loved one is dealing with aggressive, life-threatening Lyme, please move immediately to chapter eleven. It lists twenty FDA approved drugs that are not commonly used for Lyme treatment and could save your loved one's life.

Have you been told Chronic Lyme is a mental condition? If you don't know why your doctor isn't taking your symptoms seriously, we'll talk about that in chapter one.

Don't know why, after months of aggressive treatment, you still feel terrible? It's likely that you're dealing with an immune system problem, not a Lyme problem. We'll talk about Lyme and the immune system in chapter six.

Would it surprise you to learn that healing from Lyme can and should feel better? Not just at the end. Every single day you're living with Chronic Lyme you should gradually feel better. We'll talk about Lyme and the Healing Response in chapter seven.

In this book, I will tell you why you should stop doing things that make you feel wretched. Why? The process of making you feel worse with treatment is supporting the illness, not your healing. Inflaming your body with aggressive, miserable treatments defeats the purpose of the treatments. It depletes your immune system, and it creates a no-win situation for patients; either you feel terrible with the illness or you feel terrible with the treatment.

Aggressive treatments in Chronic Lyme cases may not

help more than more moderate treatments. We need to work toward lifelong treatment plans for patients with Chronic Lyme. The current model of Lyme has been a focus on a single infection or set of infections. Instead, we need to recognize that re-infection is now the new normal and cannot allow it to derail recovering patients. Creating a plan for patients so that they can continue to recover from any future infection must be our goal.

Why did I write this book?

When I finished my first book explaining the Lyme Wars, *Why Chronic Lyme Doesn't (And Does) Exist,* patients asked me what I would do myself if I had Chronic Lyme. I'd like to think I'd find a middle way, but it's a lot easier to sit on the sidelines of the Lyme Wars than to make the choices myself.

So I wrote this book from the standpoint of what I would do if I had Chronic Lyme. I will base everything I write here on the best evidence-based medical research we have.

Yes, I will also tell you what I would do personally, which has changed as I've researched. For example, at the beginning of my research the Lyme vaccine still sounded like a good idea. Now, not so much. (My current reaction is more like, "Yikes! Run away!" Since I've learned the vaccine can cause all the Lyme symptoms in some people.)

I have the great advantage of having my mind clear and my joints currently pain-free, so I don't have to struggle with the misery of Chronic Lyme while I examine my options.

For those of you who believe that only someone who currently suffers from the disease has special insight, I have also accessed the many online Lyme chat boards, examining the popular treatments from first person accounts. I also have access to and understand the herbal as well as conventional medical options. So while I don't have the illness (at least current symptoms), I do understand it.

For every person with Chronic Lyme, the journey is individualized. I hope my own journey will be helpful to you as I consider the most fruitful choice of treatments.

1 I Am Angry About Chronic Lyme

I apologize if this book seems at times to be angry. No particular person or treatment makes me angry, I'm just angry about Chronic Lyme.

I'm not just angry because the Centers of Disease Control and Prevention (CDC) continues to claim it doesn't exist. They are hurting so many people without any justification. It bothers me every day that they've taken the "just say no" position to Chronic Lyme, despite the accepted reality that between ten and twenty percent of Lyme patients may have lingering symptoms.[i] But I'm used to that head-in-the-sand mentality. It continues even though Chronic Lyme is now four times more common in the U.S. than AIDS[ii] and still the CDC thinks of it as a "subjective syndrome" because they could not locate the infectious agent to their satisfaction.[iii]

What also makes me angry is that, after forty years, we

still are no closer to fixing Chronic Lyme. We still don't have any studies that show a cure. The "Lyme literate" doctors of ILADS (International Lyme and Associated Diseases Society) are the only ones even treating Chronic Lyme. They (we, as I'm at least "semi-Lyme literate") stuff their patients full of chemical cocktails in the hopes of a cure.[iv] Why?

"The plausible idea that additional antimicrobial therapy for potentially persistent bacterial infection would foster improvement has been a touchstone of hope in the 40 years since discovery of the disease."-M.T. Melia[v]

But we live in a world where Lyme is endemic. An endemic disease is one that is always present, one which is expected to continue to be a problem indefinitely. Think of it like malaria being endemic in the tropics or gas pain being an endemic result of eating beans. Lyme being endemic means that experts no longer consider it possible that the disease will ever disappear.

In an endemic Lyme world, re-infection over time is virtually assured. So the drug cocktails will not fix the problem. What the extended drug cocktails do is speed the antibiotic resistance of Lyme. As the resistance spreads, the answer is to add more drugs. The focus on more medications makes me wonder when the "alternative medicine" crowd become the drug pushers?

I'm angry many patients treated for Chronic Lyme seem as bad as they did before treatment, and often look worse off. As we add more drugs, the side effects from those drugs also increase. But ILADS doesn't call them drug side effects. We call them a healing response, a healthy "herxing" reaction of the body's immune system.

Only in the bizarre world of Chronic Lyme does feeling terrible equal a healing response. Even cancer doctors have the honesty to admit that chemo has side effects. Losing your hair and vomiting all day is not a "healing response." It doesn't matter if you're suffering from Lyme or cancer.

In much of this book I will be talking about the shortcomings of many current Chronic Lyme treatments. Since ILADS doctors are the only ones currently treating Chronic Lyme, it may seem that all my irritation is directed at them. Let me be clear, I have the greatest respect for ILADS doctors. CDC doctors are not even trying to treat an epidemic of Chronic Lyme, so they will be ignored for much of this book. Just as the CDC doctors ignore or downplay the suffering of thousands of patients, a position I find completely inconsistent with our Hippocratic Oath to alleviate suffering. The few ILADS doctors trying to treat the Chronic Lyme epidemic deserve our gratitude even if they fall far short of a cure.

We need to move forward with a lifelong plan for Chronic Lyme patients. It can't be to call them mentally ill like the CDC and we can't expect them to eat a drug cocktail forever like ILADS. I don't have all the answers. But I know the direction we need to go, the way forward. I know it is possible to live symptom-free in our infectious world.

2 Does Chronic Lyme Even Exist?

While Lyme is a global issue, we'll be talking mostly about Lyme in the U.S. Here in the U.S. there are two groups that deal with Lyme, ILADS (International Lyme and Associated Diseases Society) and the CDC (Centers of Disease Control and Prevention). The CDC is the default group for Lyme, making up the vast majority of doctors and testing. According to the CDC, Lyme is easily tested for, easily treated, and Chronic Lyme does not exist.[vi] In comparison, ILADS considers Lyme to be harder to test for, almost impossible to treat successfully, and they are the ones primarily treating Chronic Lyme.[vii]

As you can imagine, the two groups of doctors from ILADS and the CDC don't see eye-to-eye. The reality is that both sets of doctors lack large scale, definitive studies on either Lyme testing[viii] or treatment.[ix] Neither one is truly in a position to say the other side is absolutely wrong because patients often do not present with clear symptoms.[xxi] We also lack a definitive, internationally recognized answer on whether Chronic Lyme exists.

But we should recognize now that when we discuss the symptoms and treatment of Chronic Lyme we are discussing a tiny portion of the whole.[xii] The vast majority of people who contract Lyme will not have symptoms. Those that do have symptoms will likely be made symptom-free (though they may continue to test positive for Lyme) after a month of antibiotics.

So when we discuss Chronic Lyme we are talking about the rare individual who gets symptoms and those symptoms are not resolved by a single course of antibiotics.[xiii] It is likely that these individuals are suffering from other illnesses or processes that alter their immune response to Lyme, sapping their ability to mount a sufficient defense. These are the Chronic Lyme patients.

I'm a heretic in the Lyme Wars who doesn't follow either the CDC or the ILADS playbook. I don't think strictly defined Chronic Lyme exists. If every lab test for Lyme showed a rampant infection of the Lyme spirochete in the bloodstream, none of the Lyme debate would be happening. But there is no rampant bloodstream infection. It has either been cured (the CDC viewpoint) or has gone into the cells (the ILADS viewpoint). So a narrowly defined Chronic Lyme blood infection does not exist.

BUT...though I don't believe in narrowly defined Chronic Lyme, I do think that broadly defined Chronic Lyme exists. By broadly defined, I mean a set of symptoms that may be caused by antibiotic resistance, other Lyme species,[xiv] co-infections, and/or autoimmune Lyme reactions. Including these broader factors in the definition of Chronic Lyme means we are not talking about an overwhelming blood infection by the one Lyme species the CDC recognizes as valid. We are talking about an ill-defined cluster of associated diseases that fall loosely under the Chronic Lyme umbrella.

Calling them all Chronic Lyme is the equivalent to calling every sniffle "the flu." It makes sense to laypeople, but it isn't technically correct. The Infectious Diseases Society of America (IDSA), which writes the CDC's guidelines for Lyme, gets grumpy when people misname influenza and when people talk loosely about Chronic Lyme. They prefer the term PLDS (Post-Lyme Disease Syndrome). But Chronic Lyme is shorter, and as popular in common usage as the 'flu.

Just realize we are talking about all the related infections and symptoms when we say Chronic Lyme. Recently an ILADS practitioner corrected me to say that he does not treat Chronic Lyme, he treats MSIDS (Multiple Systemic Infectious Disease Syndrome). A better name might be Chronic Tick Disease, but I realize we don't need yet another name for the illness. We need a cure.

3 What Do We Really Know About Lyme?

I will retell the story of Lyme very briefly here, with a focus on the treatments that have been used to cure it over the decades.

Once upon a time there was a rash called ECM (erythema chronica migrans) that European loggers got occasionally and which went away with antibiotics. Any antibiotic worked. Even penicillin was great. No one thought much about ECM. Occasionally someone would get really sick from it, but mostly people just lived with it.[xv]

Then in the 1970's a bunch of kids in Lyme, Connecticut got rashes and joint pains.[xvi] No one knew what caused it, but antibiotics seemed to help. Some people got better on antibiotics after years of being on them.

It was ten years before a researcher proved the Lyme outbreak was a bacteria. Over those ten years doctors treating "Lyme" tried a lot of treatments, and had a lot of successes and failures. So they became the experts in treating Lyme and the core of what became ILADS (the International Lyme and Associated Diseases Society).

Later on, the CDC (Centers of Disease Control and Prevention) tried to copy the ILADS doctors' results by giving a lot of antibiotics to people with Chronic Lyme symptoms. The CDC did not find them helpful.[xvii] So they told the ILADS doctors to stop, because the CDC claims expertise in all infectious diseases including Lyme. But the ILADS doctors said the Lyme bacteria could do clever things like hide inside the cells of the body. They said the CDC should leave them alone and kept treating.

Both sides of that argument still exist.[xviii] One side is called IDSA (Infectious Diseases Society of America) and wrote the guidelines for treating Lyme that the CDC uses. Those guidelines do not recognize long-term antibiotics as helpful for Chronic Lyme. Most doctors in the U.S. are IDSA doctors even if they don't know it.

The other side calls themselves ILADS. ILADS believes

that long-term antibiotics are still necessary and must be supported by a range of other medications to help lower the Chronic Lyme infection.[xix] Unless your doctor claims to be ILADS, they are IDSA and follow the CDC's guidelines for treating Lyme.

The CDC doesn't recognize Chronic Lyme as a legitimate disease. They think it is a mental illness or some other illness masquerading as Lyme.[xx] So patients who go to CDC doctors with symptoms that might be Chronic Lyme get treated oddly. The doctors may be reluctant to send out for Lyme testing. They may resist giving a patient antibiotics. It's because they are being told by the CDC that the disease isn't real.

ILADS doctors believe Chronic Lyme is real. They also believe it never goes away. No one ever recovers from Chronic Lyme. Even if patients have no symptoms they still have the Lyme bacteria hiding in their bodies. These bacteria form spores that cannot be killed off. So ILADS doctors treat patients with a lot of antibiotics and other drugs in an effort to bring down the numbers of these hard-to-kill bacteria. But they do not believe that patients are ever cured of Chronic Lyme. It can always come back.

Both the CDC and ILADS have tests for Chronic Lyme. They use different laboratories and read the results differently.[xxi] Both of them are certain their labs are better. But both sets of labs cannot say for sure if a patient does or does not have Chronic Lyme.[xxii]

When looking at the overall treatment for Lyme, the CDC is correct that more antibiotics don't seem to help or even be necessary.[xxiii] But in specific subgroups with continuing symptoms antibiotics might help[xxiv] and other supportive treatment is certainly necessary. That's the reality which is recognized by ILADS.[xxv] Whether more antibiotics will help in those subgroups is still open to question. But there is no question that at least some patients have a continuing set of symptoms, sometimes very severe.[xxvi]

In the world there are other Lyme researchers besides ILADS and the CDC. A big research center in Europe called the Cochrane Review has looked at what we really know about Chronic Lyme. Here is what we definitely know about Lyme based on the Cochrane Database, a European clearinghouse that analyzes all existing studies on a subject.

Cochrane on Lyme: Yes, taking Doxycycline can help.

Doxycycline treatment after a tick bite will lower your risk of getting Lyme from 2% to less than 1%.[xxvii]

Cochrane on Nerve Symptoms: We don't know if lots of antibiotics help untreated "Lyme brains."

"It is not possible to draw firm conclusions" because the studies done by any doctors (on either side of the issue) were so poorly done.[xxviii]

Cochrane on children: We don't have know the best Lyme treatment for children.

"Data is scarce and with limited quality."[xxix]

Cochrane on the CDC: The CDC guidelines are not the final word on Lyme.

"No statement can be given on quality of content and validity of recommendations"[xxx]

Cochrane on lab testing: We don't know the best way to test for Lyme.

They didn't find any unbiased studies, and the results were heterogeneous, which means they were all over the map.[xxxi]

Cochrane on Chronic Lyme: We can't say whether or not Chronic Lyme exists.

"patients may experience residual symptoms after treatment with a prevalence of approximately 28%." But those symptoms may or may not be from Lyme.[xxxii]

After forty years of dealing with Lyme we really don't know anything more than we did way back before ECM started being called Lyme. The old doctors knew that antibiotics sometimes seemed to help with the symptoms. That's still all we know for certain now. And that's using the best analyses of all existing medical studies by the world's experts.

4 Can't I Just Take Lots of Antibiotics?

When Lyme came out as a bacteria everyone thought that there was going to be an easy solution. It was just a bacteria, one that was easily killed by any antibiotic.

But Lyme has become antibiotic resistant over the years. The resistance is well-documented.[xxxiii] But neither the CDC nor ILADS doctors want to admit the current treatments for Lyme may not work in the future. The CDC thinks Lyme is easily killed, and ignores the possibility of antibiotic resistance. ILADS doctors think Lyme is impossible to kill but they want to use every possible tool they have available right now to try. Neither side wants to consider a world in which Lyme is fully resistant to all pharmaceutical drugs.

As a doctor living in a clearly endemic northeastern state

(Maine), I need to consider a reality where Lyme may become untreatable with antibiotics in my lifetime. So I will consider this as I go forward in my own research. We need solutions that will work for patients ten years from now, not just tomorrow.

A patient may have Lyme and not get better with antibiotics. When that happens it is best to rethink the diagnosis. If the patient is with a CDC doctor they will rethink the illness, come up with another diagnosis, and try other drugs.

But if the patient is with an ILADS doctor they will get more antibiotics and other drugs to still try to treat Chronic Lyme.[xxxiv] The idea is to overcome the antibiotic resistance by increasing the dosages or adding other antibiotics. Sometimes this works and the patients improve.

In other cases, patients might be better off with CDC doctors because their symptoms may never respond to any Lyme antibiotic treatment. Years of treatment, thousands of dollars of debt, and multiple side effects to their medications may not benefit them in the end.

Today many ILADS doctors recognize the futility of pounding away at Chronic Lyme with more drugs and have switched to primarily treating the co-infections that show up with Lyme. These co-infections are other diseases spread by ticks. Some of these co-infections may even have caused the patient to test positive for Lyme despite never having Lyme.[xxxv]

The co-infections include an ever-lengthening list of rarer diseases. All of them have less research available on either testing or treatments than Lyme, which means we don't have any large studies on diagnosing or treating them. Patients treated for these co-infections may feel much better. If they don't, it's hard to know if they truly had those co-infections or not. The CDC researchers have already weighed in to say that none of the co-infections even exist in the general population.[xxxvi]

The symptoms of Chronic Lyme may also be from many other diseases besides Lyme or its co-infections. Just because someone has been bitten by a tick doesn't mean his or her joint pain is from Lyme. Or that for the rest of their life every illness is a result of that bite.

In a practical medical world, the diagnosis of a disease leads to a treatment that works to cure the patient. If a diagnosis does not lead to any treatment that works to cure or even improve the symptoms of the illness, then a patient should look for a second opinion.

Many patients find the diagnosis of Chronic Lyme only after other diagnoses and treatments haven't helped. It is a blessing for them and their families when they finally get relief from their symptoms. But some patients get stuck on the Chronic Lyme diagnosis even when no Chronic Lyme treatment has worked. They forget that a diagnosis is only as useful as the resulting successful treatment. No one gets any benefit from a diagnosis without any available treatment.

5 Can't I Just Move?

In my other book, *Why Chronic Lyme Doesn't (And Does) Exist,* I tracked Lyme much farther than the northeast of the United States. Lyme disease has been found all over Europe.[xxxvii] It's also found in different areas of China.[xxxviii] Lyme disease infects people in northeastern India.[xxxix] And it's in places it shouldn't be according to the CDC, like the Caribbean and Egypt.[xl] So Lyme isn't an isolated illness confined to the northeast U.S., California, and the upper Midwest of the U.S. It is a global illness. There are no safe areas to live, and the incidence of Lyme diagnosis is consistently increasing.[xli]

The spread of Lyme is not limited to just one tick. From the beginning Lyme was spread by at least three different ticks,[xlii] one in the Northeast, one on the Pacific Coast, and a third in Europe.[xliii] It may also be spread by fleas,[xliv] mites,[xlv] biting flies,[xlvi] mosquitoes,[xlvii] [xlviii] by sex,[xlix] during pregnancy,[l] and by urine.[li] [lii] Avoiding tick bites is not going to avoid Lyme exposure.

Lyme is not a single species. There are sixteen different Lyme species. Recently the Mayo clinic found a seventeenth.[liii] We do not know if all the species are equally infectious or if they all cause the same symptoms.

The list of other diseases (co-infections) that can be spread by a tick is also always growing. Here in the U.S. we have a different list of likely co-infections than they do in Europe.

The common infections caught along with Lyme from ticks in the U.S. include Anaplasmosis, Bartonella, and Babesia. These can be tested for, but being positive for them does not prove they are causing the current symptoms, only that you had the disease at some point. With the exception of Babesia, the other diseases are treated with the same antibiotics as Lyme.[liv] So a person bitten by tick with symptoms like Lyme could be treated and have a co-infection resolve without ever knowing that's what she really had.

Remember that ticks may not be necessary to become infected. In China one of the co-infections (Anaplasma) was spread by living in the same hospital ward as an infected patient who was coughing blood. So it may not be possible to avoid getting a co-infection even if you avoid sex, pregnancy, urine, or being bitten by anything.[lv]

Readers hoping to avoid Lyme infection by living in a Lyme free area should be very concerned. It isn't possible to avoid Lyme by moving and living in a Lyme-free area because Lyme is far more prevalent than we've been told by the CDC. Anyone in a CDC recognized Lyme area has likely already been exposed to Lyme directly or indirectly. If by some miracle you haven't been exposed, you will be - regardless of the extent of your precautions.

So Should I Panic?

Panicking and increasing your precautions may actually be harmful. Taking aggressive precautions, like always taking an antibiotic after every tick bite, may not help in the long run. Using an antibiotic immediately means that the body never develops any immune response to the disease. The body assumes that an antibiotic is always going to be available. The result leaves a person more likely to respond badly to future bites.[lvi] More importantly, after taking antibiotics and partially treating Lyme a person lowers the ability of labs to accurately detect future Lyme exposure. Active, untreated Lyme can be seen clearly on labs far more easily than older, partially treated Lyme.[lvii]

Here's The Good News In A Lyme World

The overwhelming majority of those exposed to Lyme do not show symptoms. Just because you've been exposed does not mean you will get any symptoms of Lyme. And it's far less likely you will develop Chronic Lyme even if you've had Lyme symptoms.

Think of being exposed to Lyme like being exposed to a sneeze. Sneezes are full of bacteria. You may catch a cold, but you may not. And if you catch a cold, you'll most likely get well.

Other factors besides the sneeze determine how bad the cold will be. First is if you've been exposed to the bugs in the sneezed before. If you have, then you'll likely wipe out the sneeze bugs without even noticing. Next is if your immune system is up to speed: rested, relaxed, and without any other current infections to distract it. Again, most likely you never know you were infected. If your immune system isn't up to speed, then you notice some symptoms from the sneeze, maybe feeling tired. But only if you've never been exposed before, if your immune system is distracted, and if you ignore the first signs of needing to take care of yourself, will you come down with the symptoms of a cold.

Even if you get a cold, very few people who get sneezed on will develop severe symptoms like pneumonia from it. How many sneezes have you been exposed to without developing pneumonia? Think of Lyme exposure in the same way. You may be exposed to Lyme many times without ever developing symptoms, and even more often without developing Chronic Lyme.

6 Lyme And The Immune System

Most people exposed to Lyme show no symptoms. Most of those who do show symptoms get better with a short round of antibiotics. So being exposed to Lyme alone does not cause Chronic Lyme. Being exposed to Lyme and having an abnormal immune response is what causes Chronic Lyme.

What We Can Learn From Failure

Many researchers have investigated the possible autoimmune connection between Lyme and the body. Perhaps the most invested researchers are the manufacturers of the Lyme vaccine LYMErix. For those who missed the Lyme vaccine, it came and went for humans. Animals can still get vaccinated. LYMErix came on the market claiming immunity to Lyme, and left the market because some recipients said it caused the symptoms of Chronic Lyme in them. According to the FDA reports, the vaccine was only partially effective (about 50%) after multiple injections.[lviii]

As you can imagine, the manufacturer of LYMErix has a vested financial interest in proving their product did not cause Lyme symptoms in patients. So we should trust their research, because they did find that - in certain patients - their vaccine's active ingredient (OspA) did trigger an extreme immune response.

According to the manufacturer, the increased immune response was a massive increase in an immune marker called T(H)1. A T(H)1 cell is a little like Paul Revere, warning the other immune cells to be ready to defend the body. But too many of them can be like someone calling out "Fire!" in a crowded theater. Instead of being ready, the immune system panics. When it panics, the immune system can start attacking the body. It was this T(H)1 abnormal response, not the vaccine itself, that caused the immune system response and the symptoms that came with it.

A Bit Of Lyme Skin

In the manufacturer's defense, their product OspA is an

entirely dead bit of Lyme bacteria. The name stands for Outer Surface Protein A. It's a bit of the outer shell of the Lyme bacteria, like a bit of dead snake skin without the snake inside. There is no way OspA could cause a Lyme infection.

The manufacturer did select OspA because they knew it would cause an immune response. The idea was to trigger a mild immune response to the dead bit of Lyme skin. Later on, when the real Lyme infection showed up, the immune system would be prepared. It would destroy the future invader easily without any symptoms.

A Mutation

But the makers of the vaccine just weren't prepared for patients getting the vaccine who had a genetic mutation (HLA-DRB1) in their cells. Patients with this mutation have an immune system that locks onto the OspA molecule and just won't let go. Locking the immune system in high alert leads to the massive increase in T(H)1. When T(H)1 increases that much it leads to the overactive immune system attacking the body. Patients getting the vaccine who had this genetic mutation didn't just get Lyme symptoms, they developed antibiotic-resistant arthritis, the worst kind of Lyme arthritis.

So the drug manufacturer claims the over-reaction of the immune system, not their product, is to blame. The result for some patients is the same, chronic arthritis of the joints.[lix]

The manufacturer of LYMErix did not publish the initial connection between OspA and antibiotic-resistant arthritis. That connection was made by other researchers just as the vaccine was gaining acceptance.[lx] When the connection was publicized, it became part of the reason the vaccine failed and was eventually withdrawn from the market.

Zombie Lyme?

But we can perhaps thank the LYMErix manufacturer for one result of their vaccine. They clearly showed that a completely dead bit of a Lyme spirochete's outer shell can cause all the most common symptoms of Lyme arthritis in susceptible individuals. We're not talking about a whole dead Lyme spirochete bacteria. OspA is just a tiny bit of the whole. Not even the most adamant ILADS doctor would argue that the OspA piece somehow morphed itself back to life as an infectious agent. It was dead, but patients still had all the symptoms of Chronic Lyme.

The connection is particularly relevant today, because the vaccine discussion is still ongoing. Many researchers are trying to bring back the Lyme vaccine because they see it as a still-viable option for preventing the expansion of the Lyme epidemic.[lxi] But other newer research shows that OspA is also involved in carrying Lyme across the blood-brain barrier into the brain.[lxii] In other words, that same bit of Lyme skin could also cause all the nerve and brain symptoms associated with Lyme.

What Does The Mutation Do?

So the ten dollar question is: who is genetically susceptible to these bad Lyme reactions? Not just to arthritis but the most troubling antibiotic-resistant arthritis? The answer seems to be individuals who have a specific mutation in their major histocompatibility complex (MHC).

What the heck is an MHC? We know it's major, and we know it's a complex. The histocompatibility bit is another way of saying that the complex's job is to check if another cell or bacteria is friend or foe. Histo- is short for body, and compatibility is a relationship term. So the complex tells if something is compatible with your body.

An MHC is the part of the immune cell that goes looking for bacteria or viruses in the bloodstream like a kid looking for Easter candy. If the MHC grabs onto something, it presents it to the other immune cells. Think of the bloodstream as an Easter egg hunt and the MHC as the hunter. When the MHC finds a bacteria or virus, it grabs it and presents it to the other hunters and other immune cells. "Look what I found! Let's go get some more!" Soon all the other immune cells are looking for the same bacteria or viruses. It's a great way to defend the body when it works correctly.

In the case of the MHC mutation common to Chronic Lyme, (MHC class II allele DRB1*0401 for the science nerd readers like me) the MHC Easter egg hunter isn't very smart. It's not the poor thing's fault. This poor mutated MHC wasn't given a very good grabbing hand. Instead of having a magnetically charged hand like the other MHCs, this MHC has an uncharged, sticky hand. Think of it like not having a good magnetic claw in one of those old crane arcade games where you need a magnet to pick up the right toys and prizes. Instead of a working claw, you've got one with a faulty magnet that is also sticky from some kid's cotton candy. So, instead of finding other magnetic prizes (bacteria or viruses), this MHC picks up any old thing. Any bit of material floating by, like a rock, a piece of dirt, or even a piece of dead Lyme bacteria "skin" like OspA. This MHC will grab it and hold it up for everyone else in the immune system to see.

Not only does it hold it up, this sticky MHC will keep holding it up long after it should have put it down. It's like a kid at an Easter egg hunt who finds a rock and shouts to everyone else that she's found the biggest Easter egg of all! At first the other kids question her, but she sticks to her guns and keeps shouting about how pretty her Easter egg is. Pretty soon the other kids, the other immune hunter cells, are running around chasing rocks as well.

Same Mutation, Many Problems

We know this sticky MHC will grab pretty much anything it can, because it's not just known for its association with Lyme. The same MHC problem is associated with a greater risk of other autoimmune diseases including rheumatoid arthritis, type 1 diabetes, Lupus, and multiple sclerosis. This one error in the MHC can cause all sorts of problems in the body.[lxiii]

So people with severe arthritis from Chronic Lyme share the same genetic marker (MHC class II allele DRB1*0401) as people who suffer from rheumatoid arthritis.[lxiv] Perhaps a quick look at rheumatoid arthritis can give us some insight into Chronic Lyme arthritis.

What Can Happen In Rheumatoid Arthritis

Officially we don't know why people get rheumatoid arthritis either. But several bacteria may be involved. One of the bacteria that may cause rheumatoid arthritis is called Proteus mirabilis.[lxv] It lives in many people's guts happily and without any symptoms. Normally it doesn't cause problems for people.

But, in genetically susceptible people, an overgrowth of Proteus in the urinary tract can cause problems. The body's immune system sees the overgrowth of the Proteus bacteria as an attack on the body. It overreacts and mounts a very aggressive defense. In the process the body's immune system generates an enormous number of antibodies. Some of these antibodies migrate away from the person's urinary tract out to the fingers. There, in the fingers, the antibodies to the bacteria see a person's joint fluid is somehow similar in structure to the Proteus bacteria. These antibodies do what they think they were meant to do, and attack those joint structures. Antibodies to Proteus have been found in the knuckle swelling fluid of rheumatoid arthritis patients. When those patients have less Proteus growing in their guts and urinary tracts, many of them have less rheumatoid arthritis symptoms.[lxvi] But we don't see the Proteus bacteria themselves in the joints of the rheumatoid arthritis patients. We only see the immune system's antibodies to the Proteus bacteria attacking the joints.

A Chronic Lyme Comparison?

In patients with Chronic Lyme antibiotic-resistant arthritis we may see the same picture. When a person is exposed to Lyme, his or her body mounts an aggressive response. So far so good. Hopefully the antibodies will eliminate the Lyme. The person may resolve the Lyme infection without any symptoms.

But in Chronic Lyme patients these antibodies may also go looking for Lyme in the body's own tissues. If we believe the ILADS version of Chronic Lyme rather than the CDC, Lyme bacteria can enter the cells of the body and live inside. Pursuing Lyme inside its own cells could trigger the immune system just like an active Lyme bacterial infection in the bloodstream. The battle has shifted from the bloodstream to the body's own cells where it continues without ending.

Even if the Lyme bacteria don't enter the cells of the body, a genetically susceptible patient may have aggressive antibodies that could see the body's own tissues as being similar to Lyme. Something in the body's own cells could look enough like Lyme to continue to generate an immune response. So Lyme antibodies could attack their own body's tissues while trying to fight the Lyme even if no Lyme exists in those cells.

If we look at Chronic Lyme treatment in this light, taking even a cocktail of antibiotics will only help by decreasing the number of active Lyme bacteria. The symptoms of Chronic Lyme may decrease, but the underlying immune antibodies will last for months and may flare again if the immune system feels attacked - with or without more actual active Lyme infection.

Is Any Lyme Left At All?

The vaccine manufacturer of LYMErix claims that the bodies of patients with Chronic Lyme continue to attack themselves in the absence of any Lyme triggers. Chronic Lyme arthritis patients begin with Lyme DNA in their joint fluid. This Lyme DNA can include dead bits of Lyme like OspA. But in these Chronic Lyme patients a part of their own cells also looks a lot like OspA. The part of their cells that looks similar to OspA is called LFA-1 (human lymphocyte function–associated antigen-1, or specifically hLFA-1αL332–340 for the nerds among us). For these Chronic Lyme arthritis patients, OspA and LFA-1 looked enough alike to trigger an immune response to both of them.

Because part of their own cell structure looks like OspA to their immune systems, these Chronic Lyme arthritis patients still had continuing symptoms even after OspA and all other Lyme DNA were gone from their synovial joint fluid. These aren't just patients who don't have Lyme infections anymore. These are Chronic Lyme arthritis patients who didn't even have any leftover Lyme DNA in their cells. Their bodies were completely clean of Lyme down to a cellular level. But they still had the symptoms of Chronic Lyme arthritis.[lxvii]

Now, the manufacturer may not be accurate in claiming that no Lyme traces existed anywhere in these patients' bodies. But they make a convincing case for autoimmunity based on a combination of genetic susceptibility and a triggering compound, even if the triggering compound (OspA) isn't infectious on its own.

The Broader Case For Abnormal Immunity

We don't need to rely on the vaccine manufacturer to make the case for the autoimmunity of Chronic Lyme. As early as 1987 researchers found some Lyme patients had positive rheumatoid factor (similar to what is found in rheumatoid arthritis), showing that their bodies were attacking themselves.[lxviii]

The early studies of Lyme found immune cells in the arthritic joints of Lyme patients. These immune cells became irreversible solids at low temperatures (cryoglobulins), and continued to gunk up the joint long after the active Lyme infection was resolved. All the Lyme patients who continued to have arthritic symptoms also continued to have these immune cells in their joints.[lxix] But in some unlucky Lyme patients, these immune cells also remained throughout the body, leading to all sorts of other symptoms.[lxx]

So some Chronic Lyme patients continue to have symptoms despite the drug cocktails, and despite a decrease in their Lyme markers on lab tests. We know that DNA from Lyme can still be found in some patients' bodies even after they no longer have active Lyme bacteria. ILADS sees this as proof of continuing active Lyme infection, while the CDC thinks this is unimportant.

Even without the bacteria, even without the Lyme DNA in their cells, the immune antibodies to Lyme may continue to attack a patients' own tissue. CDC doctors have no explanation for what's going on.[lxxi] ILADS doctors say the Lyme has moved inside the body's own cells and we should continue to pursue it aggressively with more drugs.

Let's assume that the DNA of the Lyme bacteria does continue within the cells, either alone or in another, less active form of the bacteria. Once the genetic material -the DNA- of Lyme has integrated into a body's own cells, we are no longer discussing infection. An attack of the immune system on the body's own cells is called autoimmune disease.

But many of the treatments used by ILADS doctors are for

treating a continuous, ongoing infection. They say that people on antibiotics get better over a long time. But studies of Chronic Lyme patients show they get better over a long time with or without any more antibiotics.[lxxii] Untreated people with Chronic Lyme symptoms who never receive any antibiotics also improve over time. Over the years, even untreated people have a progressive decrease in their Lyme arthritis, etc. So the extended antibiotic treatments may be doing nothing at all.

What would be more effective is to treat Chronic Lyme patients as autoimmune patients. We should move away from the infectious model entirely as the disease continues from months to years. But neither the CDC nor ILADS has made the transition to using primarily autoimmune treatments.

7 The Herx Jerks

If Chronic Lyme is primarily autoimmune, then long-term antibiotics won't help much. But there's no harm in trying, right? Just as there's no harm in trying a cocktail of other drugs. Even if they've never been approved by the FDA for treating Lyme or shown to be effective for treating Lyme. All of these drugs might help because they affect Lyme growth in a test tube. So we guess they might help in the body. We don't know for sure, but what's the harm in trying?

ILADS doctors know that the aggressive antibiotics used on Chronic Lyme patients may cause severe reactions.[lxxiii] These are called Jarius-Herxheimer reactions (JHR), and were first noted almost a century ago in syphilis patients. Since syphilis and Lyme bacteria are both spirochetes (spiral snakelike bacteria), the assumption has been that a similar response occurs when treating both. In the Chronic Lyme community the Jarius-Herxheimer reactions are very familiar and are commonly called "herx reactions" or "herxing."

What is a typical Jarius-Herxheimer reaction? Patients may spike a fever with shaking chills and a worsening of skin rashes within a short time after getting intravenous antibiotics for syphilis or any other spirochete bacterial infection (Lyme, leptospirosis, relapsing fever).[lxxiv] In one case it came on within an hour and lasted only ten minutes.[lxxv] It usually mounts within a few hours and resolves within two days.

The Jarius-Herxheimer reaction may be severe. Patients may have seizures, their breathing may stop, they could have a stroke, and they may die.[lxxvi] All of these are documented "herxing" reactions to aggressive antibiotic treatment of syphilis. It is the reason why syphilitic patients are always hospitalized when receiving aggressive treatment for syphilis.

Patients receiving a similar treatment for Lyme are not hospitalized. The danger from the reaction is downplayed. Even the name of the reaction is shortened from a Jarius-

Herxheimer reaction to a less threatening "herxing."

A Reality Check

Let's begin with a reality check of the bigger picture of where we are when we discuss "herxing." Much of the medical establishment does not consider Chronic Lyme to be a valid diagnosis. They base their opinion on a very narrow definition of Lyme, and on a few large studies that didn't show much benefit from taking long-term antibiotics. Instead, many CDC doctors consider Chronic Lyme to be a mental condition, an obsession by the patient. When they dismiss the Chronic Lyme patients' pain and suffering, those patients quite rightly feel very angry. They are suffering, and no one is willing to help them. So naturally those patients seek out ILADS doctors.

If we then enter into the ILADS framework of Chronic Lyme, the ILADS doctors see it as a very real, very tricky disease. Patients meeting with an ILADS doctor feel listened to, cared for, and feel much better that someone is taking them seriously. So far, ILADS wins hands down for compassion and good doctoring. They also win for the placebo response.

The placebo response should not be confused with the placebo effect. A placebo effect is a defined by taking a sugar pill and it having have the same results as a drug. But over the years the placebo effect has dropped off to where it no longer shows up as a significant effect.[lxxvii] What has grown over time is the placebo response based on the caring of a doctor who listens and responds with kindness. The cascade of hormones released by the stress reduction, the rekindling of hope, has a profoundly positive effect on the human body. The placebo response is so powerful it can outperform the effect of even the strongest drugs.[lxxviii] So we should recognize that ILADS doctors can have a healing benefit even before they begin treating for Chronic Lyme.

Within the ILADS framework, it's very hard to test for Lyme. If we believe that the bacteria can leave the blood stream, then what good is a blood test? So most ILADS doctors will treat for Lyme without a positive test, based only on the symptoms. Looking at those symptoms, a range of other illnesses could also be involved. But the reason for beginning Lyme treatment is that a trial will either improve the patient's condition or it will not.

Realize at this point we've left all lab markers to the side.

There is no objective reason to treat for Lyme except that the patient's symptoms fall within the broad range of those that could be caused by Lyme. So the only marker of success, and the only proof that it is in fact Lyme that we're treating, is if the patient improves with treatment.

A Case Study

I've done this trial myself, offering a patient a trial of doxycycline when her pain resisted all other efforts to improve it. Within two days she was pain-free. Off the doxycycline her pain returned. That was a trial-and-error test for Lyme that came back positive because the patient improved with the treatment.

What if the patient, rather than improving on doxycycline, said it had no effect? The reasonable assumption would be that she didn't have Lyme. She might, but it wasn't improved by the basic treatment. Lacking any history of a tick bite, I would have moved on to other possible diagnoses and treatments that might benefit her pain. This process of trial-and-error, finding what will work for a patient and make them better, is the empirical practice of medicine. It's always better to have a large study that says a treatment probably works, but we lack those studies in many areas of medicine. So trial-and-error is often what we have to rely on.

Let's say the patient called me in two days and told me that her pain was much worse on the doxycycline. I would tell her to stop taking the doxycycline, and do what I could to decrease her symptoms. My immediate response would be based on the very real possibility that the doxycycline was causing her pain to worsen. Since making the patient's pain worse is not my goal, stopping the drug is the only reasonable solution. If her pain resolved in a day or two off the medication, we would assume that she was allergic to the drug. A drug allergy is just medicalese for "she reacts badly to doxycycline."

When Bad Becomes Good

But, as anyone who reads the online Chronic Lyme chat boards will shout, that bad reaction to doxycycline was actually a healing response. My patient was "herxing," getting better because she was feeling worse and having more symptoms. I should have explained "herxing" to her, kept her on the medication, and encouraged her to even up the dosage to increase the pain. Only by going through that pain could she truly get better from Lyme, truly eradicate the spirochete bacteria from her body.

Accepting for the moment the "herxing" healing response idea at face value, at what point would it be too much? If a patient's pain is worsened by the treatment, I've already done the exact opposite of what she paid me to do: relieve her pain. How long should I allow her to be in agony before I call off this so-called healing response?

What if my patient starts dehydrating from the pain and needs to be hospitalized? Should I still demand she continue her healing response? And what am I basing my assumption on? My patient had no tick history, her symptoms were arthritis. I did no lab work to confirm she had Lyme, and I had no evidence that the treatment is not an allergic response. In other words, at what point does the assumption of worsening symptoms being good become bad for the patient?

Bad Is Bad For Everyone

Since the work of ILADs doctors on Chronic Lyme is being done without the support of much of the medical profession, I would argue that the only reasonable standard of care within ILADS is that the patient must improve on the treatment. A single hospitalization from a "healing response" places all ILADS doctors in a more precarious position. It infuriates the CDC doctors and puts the ability to continue treatment for all Chronic Lyme at risk.[lxxix]

Any time an ILADS doctor disregards a patient's suffering as a "healing response" he or she should be aware that of the disconnect. At that moment, the ILADS doctors are doing the same thing CDC doctors do when they tell a Chronic Lyme patient to seek mental health counseling. The effect is the same. Rather than working to lessen the suffering, the doctor is "turfing it out" either to mental illness or to an overactive immune system's healing response.

For patients, the idea of a healing response feels more tolerable than being told they are crazy. So for a time, Chronic Lyme patients will hold to the ILADS treatment regardless of the agony. But if the "herxing" goes beyond their pain tolerance and they have to stop treatment, the results are bad. In addition to their original pain and suffering, Chronic Lyme sufferers are left with a feeling of failure. "If only I could have held on, I would be well now," they think. Rather than continuing to work toward their own healing, many Chronic Lyme patients give up and simply live with the pain and disability. They feel they've failed their caring ILADS doctors and themselves, so they live with both pain and shame.

The patients who fail to tolerate he regime of antibiotics are those who are the most reactive. They are the most vulnerable to both the inflammatory response to Lyme and the side effects of too much medication. So the most ill, most vulnerable Chronic Lyme patients are the most likely to face "herxing" failure.

But the failure is on the part of the physician who placed the illusion of eradication before the patients. The reality is that patients will need to live with the possibility of Chronic Lyme returning for the rest of their lives. Even if the existing Lyme was truly eradicated from the body, another tick bite could re-introduce Lyme and start the process all over again.

No one is served by pushing patients beyond their limits in the pursuit of an imaginary goal. ILADS doctors can fall into the trap of being Don Quixote, tilting at Lyme windmills while galloping over the bodies of their suffering patients. We all need to focus instead on improving every life, every day, and move away from the goal of total Lyme eradication.

When Poisoning Becomes Healing

The online chat room discussion of the Jarius-Herxheimer reaction in Lyme can be disturbing. Without an initial worsening of symptoms, many Chronic Lyme sufferers don't think a treatment is working. Moreover, they describe "herxing" for weeks on toxic pharmaceuticals whose common side effects include tendon rupture and temporary blindness.

What does this online "herxing" involve? Oh, nothing more than the signs of septic shock, including possible convulsions, stroke, and death. To be blase about side effects that include possible death makes me feel like I've entered an *Alice In Wonderland* topsy-turvy world. Recently I met a happy Chronic Lyme near-corpse who sauntered up to let me know that he's been, "Herxing like crazy but I think we've almost got the Lyme."

Let me be clear. If the treatment for Chronic Lyme requires me to experience perpetual "herxing," which to me appears to be a cavalier description of various stages of septic shock, I have little or no interest. Having had colon cancer, I know about chemotherapy, but I have no delusions that the side effects are "good for me." Claiming that nearly killing patients is necessary in the hopes of saving them is the area of experimental oncologists, not outpatient ILADS doctors.

If an ILADS doctor knows that the majority of his or her patients will experience symptoms so severe that they may convulse, have a stroke, or die, how is it compatible with their own ethical standards to treat those patients as outpatient visits? "Go home and take all these pills. You might need to call for an ambulance later on, but never mind that." Just carry on despite your body shutting down?

Of course, it's not the ILADS doctors to blame for the online obsession with "herxing" by Chronic Lyme sufferers. But ILADS doctors support an attitude among Chronic Lyme sufferers that suffering is necessary to heal. The Chronic Lyme patients online then use that same logic to justify the most horrendous and foolish treatments imaginable (see next chapter).

When Feeling Good Becomes Bad

When you have no studies to back something up, at least you want to know that it makes you feel better. At least that is the placebo effect in action.

But in the Chronic Lyme chat rooms, that which makes you feel truly terrible, really at death's door, means you're getting much better. Bring back the heavy metals (they have, silver is very popular), bring back the purgatives (salt diarrhea, anyone?) bring back everything painful and terrible, every single wrecked remedy from the last two hundred years. I'm frankly surprised no one has thought to just rub their skin raw and squeeze lemon juice on it. God help me, that's probably the next treatment for Chronic Lyme skin disease.

The Origins Of Herxing

The justification for allowing, and even welcoming, the Jarius-Herxheimer reaction is that the antibiotics or other treatments are massively killing off the Lyme bacteria. As they die in droves, the Lyme bacteria release endotoxins. These endotoxins cause the symptoms of fever, etc. The more effective the treatment, the bigger the Lyme bacteria die-off. The larger the die-off, the more endotoxins released, and the worse the patient feels. As a result, many Chronic Lyme patients associate feeling really terrible with a really successful treatment. The worse they feel, the more Lyme bacteria are dying, and the more effective the treatment must be.

When you look up the Jarius-Herxheimer reaction in the medical literature, you see it discussed as a reaction to intravenous penicillin in the treatment of syphilis. There is no Lyme research showing endotoxin release. So ILADS doctors are basing the Lyme "herxing" theory on previous syphilis research mentioning possible endotoxin release. The assumption is that both syphilis and Lyme bacteria are spirochetes. So both would release endotoxins when they died.

The explanation given to patients in Chronic Lyme circles is that the dying Lyme spirochetes release toxins that cause the symptoms. Just like in syphilis.

Where Are The Endotoxins?

But syphilis research no longer supports the idea of endotoxin release from bacterial die-off. Multiple studies show no build up of endotoxins in the blood of either animal[lxxx] or human patients[lxxxi] with syphilis during a Jarius-Herxheimer reaction. We don't know for certain what causes the massive reaction, but it may be related to having multiple illnesses simultaneously (as with AIDS patients who also have syphilis co-infections). The Jarius-Herxheimer reaction normally occurs rapidly and fiercely shortly after the introduction of penicillin, resolving in a few hours or less than a day.

Instead of the release of endotoxins, what was found in syphilis patients on antibiotics experiencing a Jarius-Herxheimer reaction was a massive immune response. It looked similar to systemic septic shock.[lxxxii] In systemic septic shock the body is so full of invading bacteria it cannot protect itself. So the immune system panics, destroying the body's tissues in an effort to rid itself of the intruder. The immune system will try to kill the invader even if it kills the body in the process.

If we are blaming endotoxins for the Jarius-Herxheimer reactions of Lyme patients, we have no proof that Lyme produces these endotoxins. Our reliance on previous syphilis research is flawed. Instead, we have syphilis studies that clearly show endotoxins are not involved.

Do The Treatments "Jumpstart" The Immune System?

But do the antibiotics or other treatments cause the body to suddenly recognize the invading Lyme bacteria and mount the Jarius-Herxheimer response? Are we missing when the endotoxins are released or do they break down in the body too quickly to see? Is this a healing response even if we didn't have the correct cause?[lxxxiii] Not likely.

The first Jarius-Herxheimer reactions were noted when syphilis patients were given large doses of mercury to kill their syphilis.[lxxxiv] Mercury is a heavy metal poison, not an antibiotic.

Any ILADS doctor who says massive doses of mercury cause a healing response needs to get back in his or her time machine and return to the 1800's. Today we treat much lower accidental exposures to mercury as life-threatening environmental pollutants. A "Jarius-Herxheimer response" to a mercury exposure today would be classified as an environmental poisoning and would be treated acutely by chelating out the mercury as fast as possible. The symptoms would be seen as a cause for a class action lawsuit, not a celebration of healing detoxification.

Is "Herxing" Somehow Healthy?

But perhaps the antibiotics or other treatments are still doing something positive in Chronic Lyme patients by boosting their immune systems? Isn't the strong Jarius-Herxheimer response somehow healthy in the absence of mercury poisoning? Unlikely.

Jarius-Herxheimer reactions are also seen in patients with Leukemia. Leukemia involves the massive overgrowth of a cancerous immune system. During the acute phase of the illness, patients are hospitalized because the immune system has begun to attack the body. It shows all the classic "herxing" symptoms.[lxxxv] The Jarius-Herxheimer response is the definition of an unhealthy overactive immune response.

How Do We Prevent "Herxing?"

When testing for how to minimize the Jarius-Herxheimer reactions in syphilitic patients, researchers found that blocking an immune system response (TNF-alpha) greatly lowered the level of the reaction. Patients receiving the TNF immune blocker had half as many Jarius-Herxheimer reactions. The reactions were also much less severe.[lxxxvi]

Would all Lyme patients benefit from an immune blocker during acute antibiotic treatment? Not necessarily, as increased levels of body fat make patients less responsive.[lxxxvii] But the same TNF immune response has been found elevated in animal studies of Lyme arthritis.[lxxxviii] Taking a TNF immune blocker for other diseases is very effective at blocking the immune response to Lyme. It may even mask the symptoms of an acute Lyme infection until it becomes very severe.[lxxxix]

A Paradigm Shift

So "herxing" is entirely an immune system response rather than an endotoxin response to a bacterial die-off. It corresponds to being poisoned by a drug, not getting healthier. We need a paradigm shift within the treatment of Chronic Lyme to deny that there is ever a justified "herxing" response. All that is happening are severe drug side effects that are putting patients' lives at risk.

How common is the "herxing" response in Lyme patients? One study found that ten percent of patients experienced the reaction.[xc] That response rate is much lower than in relapsing fever, another tick based co-infection that can appear as a false positive for Lyme on laboratory tests.

In a study of relapsing fever, all the patients experienced "herxing" on antibiotics.[xci] Patients with nervous system syphilis fell somewhere in between. In studies of severe syphilis in both humans[xcii] and animals,[xciii] almost eighty percent of both experienced "herxing" in response to penicillin infusions. So doctors should expect "herxing" side effects when giving intravenous antibiotics and do so only in hospital settings. Instead, Chronic Lyme patients are commonly treated as outpatients, which puts them at risk of poorer outcomes.

An End To A Casual "Herxing" Response

What is amazing is not that "herxing" is commonplace. It's that the process is considered so carelessly by Chronic Lyme doctors and patients. Any other drug side effect that included possible death is taken extremely seriously by everyone. But patients may "herx" for weeks as outpatients without complaint.

The same group of doctors who might lecture against the ills of drug polypharmacy (taking five or more drugs at a time) will happily give nine drugs for Chronic Lyme. When patients arrive with new side effects from the drugs they are "herxing." Instead of stopping the drugs because of side effects, the patients may receive more of the same drug to increase the "herxing."

Even one Chronic Lyme patient who "herxes" until she dies is unacceptable.[xciv] The idea that patients need to feel worse to feel better is very questionable. Many ILADS doctors have realized this and no longer use aggressive treatments.

"Slow and steady" is the mantra for a chronic disease. Even if patients are miraculously cured by aggressive treatment, their chances of being exposed again are high.[xcv] The goal needs to be continual improvement of the quality of life. "Herxing" has no place in that framework.

A Reality Check

I realize that I've just stepped on the sacred cow of "herxing" being good for many of you. I haven't just stepped on it, I've run it over with a truck and backed up to finish the job. There is a process called a healing response that comes from within the body in response to a viral or bacterial infection. But that response is well known to all of us: fever, chills, and hopefully rapid resolution. The current concept of "herxing" is a perversion of that response, a corruption of what should be clearly the body throwing off an infection. Even the true healing response should be minimized if it causes pain and distress. Giving supportive care and minimizing suffering are expected at all times, in all illnesses.

8 Barking Up The Wrong Tree

The internet provides thirteen million results for Chronic Lyme treatments. Once we leave the world of CDC and ILADS doctors the next treatment we try may be determined by our chance encounters from a web search. There are so many products and plans that claim cures for Chronic Lyme we could literally spend the rest of our lives trying one a day and never run out of options.

If we use the idea of improving the patients' life rather than "herxing" as a goal, at least we have a baseline for when to stop a treatment. But how do we know which treatments to even try? If we look at the basis for different online treatments, it shouldn't be difficult to see that many treatments do not meet the goals of both strengthening the patient and modifying the immune response.

The Internet "Cures"

Rather than start searching randomly, I found a book that compiled what the author said were the top treatments from the internet. After reading it I privately renamed it "Ten Random And Possibly Harmful Things That Don't Really Treat Lyme." So I have decided to avoid mentioning the author's name and book title if I can in the hopes of dissuading any of you to read the book. I also want you to understand the author is just one of hundreds of people who will likely mislead you into distracting and possibly harmful treatment choices for Chronic Lyme.[xcvi]

The author of this random collection permanently earned my dislike because of the focus on “herxing” as the only way to tell if a treatment is working. I suppose I should be happy the author did not discover the older research on mercury and herxing. Otherwise the book might have endorsed drinking the old mercury thermometers to get a really good "herx" going.

While the author of "Ten Random Things" is not a doctor, an ILADS doctor wrote a preface to his book. The doctor is a Lyme treating psychiatrist most famous for almost shooting one of his son's underage friends. But his endorsement of the author is still troubling because it lends credibility to what is otherwise an incredible list of treatments: rife machines, detoxifications, enzymes, magnesium, lithium, the Marshall Protocol, salt and vitamin C binges, CoQ10, Mangosteen, and pulsed antibiotics.

If it sounds like a list of what you'd find if you cleaned out a Naturopathic Doctor's dusty old back clinical cabinet, you wouldn't be far off. I can imagine a frustrated ILADS doctor saying to a patient: "Here, dump all these in a box and try them one at a time. Something is bound to work." That's likely to do you about as much good.

There are some things on the random list that I don't have difficulty with as supplements or treatments, but which aren't known to treat Lyme. Things like magnesium and enzymes may or may not affect Lyme symptoms. Detoxification for a week or two is generally a nice thing to do, though I would argue that simply avoiding things like alcohol and desserts more regularly throughout the year would do more good for Chronic Lyme patients over the long-term.

Other things on the list are possibly harmful, but could

possibly be done well. Lithium is a treatment for mental illness, and it is known to damage the kidneys over time. The Lithium orotate version of lithium is supposedly more mild, but we don't have human studies to support that idea.[xcvii] Salt and vitamin C are both reasonable substances, but are recommended online by Chronic Lyme patients in toxic doses for self-treatment. Mangosteen, CoQ10, and Rife machines all might be helpful for chronic illness. But none of these things are specific to Lyme treatment. They fall into the "generally might be good for chronic illness" grab bag of treatments that extends to thousands of other supplements and treatments.

The one treatment that I might even consider for Chronic Lyme is pulsed antibiotics because it sounds like a good idea at first glance. Except that pulsed is another word for stopping and starting the same antibiotics. One thing we've learned about antibiotics is that if you give any bacteria a break, it will grow resistant. So pulsed antibiotics are not an option. Rotating antibiotics might be, but that does not necessitate a break between doses. If we're rotating antibiotics, the most broad-spectrum versions would be antibiotic plants that block Lyme growth, not the prescription drug versions that act on only one specific bacterial weakness. So I wouldn't consider pulsed antibiotics, I'd consider rotating antibiotic plants. Not really the same thing at all.

The author of "Random Lyme Stuff" is quite adamant that some antibiotics (the penicillins) “just make Lyme worse." I assume this is based on his understanding of ILADS doctors' comments disparaging different common antibiotics. However, there is no evidence this is the case. People taking those antibiotics for Lyme in research studies got better. That’s why they were prescribed and continue to be prescribed. The author is claiming that something is making you worse that makes you feel better. It causes many patients' symptoms to go away and never return. In lab tests the antibiotics show that they are getting rid of the Lyme spirochetes. So claiming that helping antibiotics are making you worse feels bizarre. The claim only makes sense if you live in a topsy-turvy "herxing" world where only the things that make you feel worse really make you better.

Marshalling Bad Choices Into A Protocol

The second treatment of the "Random Lyme Treatments I

Wouldn't Try If You Paid Me" is listed as the Marshall Protocol, which meets the criteria for a great "herxing" treatment and a really lousy choice for getting rid of Lyme. I have selected it for particular exploration because it ties back into some of the core ideas of ILADS in treating Chronic Lyme, including why some antibiotics are supposed to make Lyme worse..

The Marshal Protocol is the creation of one man, Trevor Marshall. It's not clear from the chapter in the "Random Lyme" book that Trevor Marshall has a PhD in Biomedical Engineering, not medicine. Marshall decided all on his own that Vitamin D was upsetting his immune system. He claims to have cured his own autoimmune illness (sarcoidosis, not Lyme) by lowering his vitamin D levels.

Marshall's Protocol lowers Vitamin D by avoiding all the foods that contain it. He asks patients to even take a prescription cholesterol lowering medication only for its side effect of lowering vitamin D levels. The protocol requires patients to avoid any and all sun exposure. In other words, become a vampire.

The treatment is so bad even alternative health guru Dr. Mercola took the time to warn his readers against it.[xcviii]

Anyone even considering a vampiric lifestyle should consider that the common signs of low Vitamin D levels overlap with fibromyalgia, chronic fatigue, and even depression (all common Chronic Lyme complaints as well). But the major side effect could be a loss of bone growth, leading to future fractures.[xcix]

Dr. Mattman's Research on Lyme

How did this Marshall Protocol treatment come about? It's useful to follow the logical steps Trevor Marshall did because they lead back to the heart of Chronic Lyme.

Trevor Marshall supposedly made up his protocol and cured his own sarcoidosis based on the work of Lida Mattman, who revolutionized infectious disease according to the "Random Lyme" author. She also, according to herbalist Stephen Buhner of *Healing Lyme* found out that multiple sclerosis was caused by Lyme spirochetes. (*Healing Lyme*, p. 47)

When we have several Chronic Lyme authors referencing the same researcher, we should learn more about her. Dr. Lida Mattman has a master's degree in virology and a Ph.D. in Immunology from Yale University. According to the authors, Mattman was a Nobel nominee for the 1998 Prize in medicine. It is impossible to know for certain since the Nobel Prize committee does not disclose the names of nominees until fifty years after the nominations.

Looking at Mattman's medline publications on Pubmed, we find a number of studies from the 1950s. Ah, here's the study that launched the Marshall Protocol. Under LH Mattman, a single small study discussing the existence of cell wall deficient forms of bacteria in sarcoidosis.[c] That's the basis of Marshall's entire Protocol. If you just read Mattman's study, she shows that wall-less forms of a bacteria were only found in sarcoidosis patients. Almost all of her twenty patients had them and none of her controls had any of these wall-less bacteria that she compares to tuberculosis. So it seems pretty clear that these wall-less bacteria might well cause sarcoidosis. So Trevor Marshall can be perhaps forgiven his thought that his illness was caused by wall-less bacteria. Of course, he ran with this study all the way to a Vitamin D free lifestyle, but at least he had a basis.

Or did he? If Marshall had looked a bit further, he might have found other wall-less bacteria research, on almost two hundred sarcoidosis patients, that found an almost equal number of these wall-less forms of bacteria in both the patients and the "healthy" controls.[ci] Mattman's research was only preliminary, and was not replicated in larger studies. Other, symptom-free individuals without sarcoidosis also have these wall-less bacteria. The basis of Marshall's Protocol falls apart under scrutiny (but that won't prevent hundreds of people from trying it - just in case it might work).

But perhaps these wall-less bacteria do form the basis of ongoing infection in the body? If this sounds very familiar from Chronic Lyme disease literature, it should. Dr. Lida Mattman also wrote a textbook that forms much of the basis of ILADS discussion about Chronic Lyme, *Cell Wall Deficient Forms*. It's a fascinating book, with sections entitled things like, "Snail Juice Induces Cell Wall Deficiency." In the textbook Mattman talks about all sorts of medical diseases caused by wall-less bacteria. One of the least lethal of these is Lyme. Now that the textbook is in its third edition, many of the chapter headings have been changed, but I trust that Dr. Mattman has remained true to her focus on wall-less bacterial forms causing much of the disease and havoc in the world.

ILADS doctors have used Mattman's work to say that the wall-less form of Lyme bacteria is caused by "the wrong kind of antibiotics." It's the basis for the claim that "some antibiotics are bad for you even if they make you feel better." The assumption is that the wall-less forms of Lyme are able to avoid being killed by any future antibiotics and will continue to maintain active Lyme infection.

But other researchers besides Dr. Mattman have looked at the disease-causing ability of these wall-less bacterial forms. Lyme is not unique in the production of these forms, as the wall-blocking antibiotics (penicillins and others) can generate wall-less forms from many different bacteria.[cii] The wall-less state is a throwback to an earlier bacterial evolutionary development, a precursor of the more virulent and protected walled state.[ciii] While a convincing case can be made for the possible involvement of wall-less forms of various bacteria in the persistent illness of some immune-compromised patients,[civ] other researchers have concluded that the wall-less forms are not a major cause of disease.[cv]

In Chronic Lyme patients, the non-spirochete, wall-less or spore forms have not been shown to actively cause disease.[cvi]

If the wall-less forms of Lyme are lying dormant, this would be in contrast to other wall-less bacteria, who cause active infection when they exist in sufficient quantities.[cvii] Lyme is not unique in its wall-less form, wall-less forms are typically less virulent, and if they exist in sufficient quantities they cause active, easily seen and treatable infections.

In the same textbook, Dr. Mattman ties multiple sclerosis to spirochetes. She also says Lou Gehrig's Disease (ALS) could be caused by Lyme.

These are fairly dramatic claims from a medical standpoint and it is worth looking at Dr. Mattman's logical steps to come to these conclusions. Unlike Chronic Lyme patients, ALS patients lack any antibodies to Lyme bacteria. But this does not disprove Dr. Mattman's assertion. She notes that many Lyme patients also lack antibodies to Lyme bacteria. While this may be true, it does not in any way prove a connection between ALS and Lyme disease. If the only criteria for connecting an illness to Lyme is a lack of antibodies, then most illnesses in the world meet that criteria.

It is not my purpose to question Dr. Mattman's genius. But I would question the wholesale application of her microscopic discoveries of wall-less bacterial forms to the extremely aggressive treatment of Chronic Lyme patients to attempt to rid the body entirely of these forms. As a reader, Dr. Mattman's textbook felt more one-sided rather than objectively discussing the research without an underlying agenda.

Beyond Dr. Mattman's work, the treatment protocols within ILADS for Chronic Lyme tend to be based solely on test tube trials of what kills the spirochete, without any human research. Yes, it is difficult to fund human research trials when most of your CDC colleagues refuse to acknowledge the existence of the illness. But depending solely on test tube trials and asking patients to put their lives in our hands must involve a great deal of humility and the acknowledgement that we could easily be wrong. Re-examining Dr. Mattman's work and realizing that it also justifies the Marshall Protocol should give any ILADS doctor pause.

Herbs

If you read Stephen Buhner's *Healing Lyme,* it paints a truly terrifying picture of Chronic Lyme. Lyme in Buhner's world is passed by saliva. The only real treatments are his recommended herbs taken by the ounce daily for months. From his book, we're left with the sense that these powerful, wonderful herbs will solve all our problems if we can just take them all.

Since Buhner's protocol is well-known and the most likely source of an ongoing lifelong treatment, we'll go through it in some detail later on in the book. But I want to take a moment now to discourage anyone from assuming Buhner believes for an instant that one size fits all, that one treatment will work for all patients. He is adamantly against that, and says as much in his several books.

Fast forward to Dr. Lou Rawls' online supplement protocol. Dr. Rawls claims he takes everything from Buhner. But clearly his marketing budget is much greater than Buhner's. Lou Rawls is an M.D. who got Chronic Lyme. Rawls cured his own chronic Lyme, and markets Buhner's protocol as a set of one-size-fits-all pills.[cviii] The same doses for a small woman and an obese man. Just plop your money down, swallow the pills in the prescribed dose, and watch your Lyme disappear.

As a doctor, Rawls would never prescribe the same dose of any pharmaceutical drug to all his different patients. But with the magic of herbs nothing like body weight, co-existing illnesses, or age seem to affect how much Dr. Rawls thinks patients need to take. If I sound less than excited, it's because I see the same combination of disregard for the power of herbs combined with too-broad claims every day. The last thing Chronic Lyme folks need in another cure-all plan based on magical thinking.

Stephen Buhner does not endorse Rawls' protocol. Buhner and his partner do the work daily of individualizing an herbal protocol for different patients. It's time consuming, careful work. My sense is that Dr. Rawls would rather be out kayaking than treating patients, at least that's what his marketing suggests. But there is no shortcut to healing. Rawls is shortchanging Buhner's work when he stopped being a doctor and started just selling supplements.

Homeopathics

There are also homeopathic sites that claim a one-size-fits-all model for Chronic Lyme treatment. One site tells us that using Ledum palustre for the tick bite, followed up by a rare homeopathic (aurum arsenicum) will cure most Lyme cases.[cix]

While I believe that the particular homeopath making

these suggestions has the best of intentions, others marketing homeopathics may not. One of my patients came to me complaining about side effects from a massive, lengthy round of very high potency homeopathics. What was most disturbing is that she had no Lyme symptoms when she began the plan. She was just taking the remedies to prevent future symptoms. Now she had symptoms from taking a treatment that was supposed to prevent her from ever having those symptoms. It was a bit like having someone come in for vomiting after taking a medication to prevent future vomiting. The treatment was worse than nothing at all.

When I looked into the treatment, I found a disturbingly normal state of affairs. The practitioner had taken no training in what she was prescribing. Instead, she'd been treated herself and was following what had been passed down to her from another practitioner. The medication was sold by a company, but they didn't make the homeopathics themselves. Another manufacturer was responsible. There is little FDA oversight of these products because none of these products are marketed as "diagnosing or treating disease." Such is the wild west of the alternative medical world.

I'm not someone who give up easily, so I did what the prescribing doctor should have done when the first signs of side effects showed up. After writing to the company, I spent a half-hour talking with the head doctor who formulated the product. He was aghast that his formula was being used as a preventative, saying it was only to be used by patients already experiencing severe symptoms. After we talked, he came up with a possible solution and promised to reach out to the practitioner to educate her in how the formula was supposed to be used. The company had sponsored several local seminars for practitioners, but evidently she had not attended. I told him I was very impressed by the power of his product even if it was from the side effects. I would even consider using it if I had severe symptoms. The point is that even good products from reputable companies can be misused to harm patients.

Crazy New Treatments

This month's alternative news includes two new treatments for Chronic Lyme, bee venom therapy and hyperthermia. Yes, you too can be stung by bees while suffering brain damaging heat.

The bee venom therapy was effective short-term for a single Lyme patient who eventually found that she had a co-infection and moved on to more antibiotics.[cx] But it was still being recommended in the article based on that single testimonial.

With the hyperthermia treatments, which reached such a high temperature that they exceeded the NIH's recommended panic level for a fever, the patient said she experienced some relief of symptoms. So now that patient promotes hyperthermia treatments as her job. Prospective patients can either fly to Germany to get fried or, more cheaply, learn how to generate heat stroke all on their own. The body temperatures are the same, as are the possible side effects of convulsions and death.[cxi]

If this month's treatment offerings show the new baseline of Chronic Lyme treatments, my goal for this book moves away from the need to find a cure or even a reasonable treatment for Chronic Lyme. I need to simply redirect Chronic Lyme sufferers away from potentially fatal prospective treatments. Perhaps I should simply list the hundreds of options that are simple, affordable, and non-lethal. Will they work? Perhaps, perhaps not. But they won't leave you confused, broke, or dead. Not a very high bar to reach.

Some of you will doubtless want such a list, even though it's not as useful as you might think. Start with the two thousand homeopathic remedies, add in all the kitchen spices, and then put that together with any number of gentle mind/body therapies. All of these would likely be less potentially harmful than injecting venom in high heat.

I know some of you are still so excited to drink Miracle treatment X to kill off your Chronic Lyme that you'll ignore my advice. So let me ground you with a reality check called babesia.

Babesia

While Lyme as an infectious agent is at least likely, one of its co-infections, Babesia, has been ignored by the larger medical community.

Babesia strikes hard at the heart muscle. Researchers monitoring pregnant mothers in endemic Lyme areas found no birth defects from Lyme but they did find an increase in heart muscle problems in babies.[cxii] Even the CDC says separate antibiotics are needed to treat Babesia. Testing for

Babesia can be difficult, and patients may have Babesia for years without symptoms. The U.S. blood supply is currently not tested for Babesia, so even patients in non-endemic areas could get Babesia from a blood transfusion. And this is the CDC's take on Babesia.[cxiii]

A study of Chronic Lyme patients found that half of them were really experiencing the symptoms of a Babesia co-infection.[cxiv] Other authorities say the co-infection rate with Lyme is around ten percent.[cxv] Here in the northeast of the U.S. the infection rate of our white-footed mouse population is very high. We would suspect our Babesia infection rate to be well above ten percent of those with Chronic Lyme.

So before you reach for online miracle treatment X to finally kill off that persistent Lyme spirochete, do remember Babesia.[cxvi] Yes, even if you've been treated for it with antibiotics, etc. A significant percentage of patients continue to have at least low-grade Babesia after treatment and the illness can be deadly.[cxvii] Treating Babesia correctly may involve hospitalization or at least anti-malarial medication. Finding Babesia involves getting blood work done well. A good lab technician should be able to see Babesia within the red blood cells.

My point is not that all of you have Babesia. It is that chasing crazy random Chronic Lyme "cures" is, at best, a waste of time and money. It is very likely a dangerous, possibly life-threatening distraction from finding the treatments that will improve your health.

So the next time you have an urge to consult "Dr. google," remember "he" doesn't have a medical license and "he's" probably been drinking. So take all that online advice the same way you would from a drunk at a bar. It's good for a laugh, but please don't bet your life on it.

9 Living With Lyme

Let's summarize the reality of Lyme in the 21st Century. Think of it as you can't win, you can't break even, and you can't get out of the game.

You Can't Win

Avoiding Lyme over a lifetime in an endemic area is a virtual impossibility even if we believe the CDC's version of how difficult it is to catch. At some point we're all going to get bitten. You can't win.

You Can't Break Even

Once we've been bitten and exposed to Lyme our bodies will react. Either we will react normally or abnormally. We don't know what the reaction will be until it happens. If we get bitten again, later on, we may react differently. You can't break even and always hope for the same response.

You Can't Get Out Of The Game

If we've been bitten and we react abnormally there is no sure cure. None of the doctors treating Chronic Lyme can tell us that we'll never have a relapse or be exposed again in the future. You can't get out of the game.

If It Seems Hopeless

I chose the same description for Lyme as the laws of energy. You can't get energy from nothing (you can't win). Energy dissipates (you can't break even). And energy is

erved (you can't get out of the game).

e energy every day. It's the fuel for your body,

house. Energy is how this book was

to read right now. Just because

planet is scary doesn't

without energy. We

what we know to help

The Way Out

Apply those same three laws to our own immune system's response to Lyme. Your immune system needs constant nutrition, rest, and awareness (you can't win by ignoring it). The immune system is going to do odd things over time. Maybe you'll get an allergy to food or pollen that you didn't have before. Your immune system is not static, it is reactive (you can't break even and pretend nothing will ever change). It's not an option to shut down your immune system for a few days. Without your immune system, you will be dead in a couple of days (you can't get out of the game).

Things Can Get Better

Let's go back to the second step. Once we've been bitten and exposed to Lyme our bodies will react. That reaction can change. It can get dramatically worse. But that means it ca[illegible] also get dramatically better. If we change our focus f[illegible] avoiding Lyme entirely to avoiding the serious side eff[illegible] Lyme then a whole range of possibilities opens up.

What if the goal of living in an endemic Lyme world is not to avoid exposure but to avoid reaction? Is this possible?

Yes. Most people exposed to Lyme do not react. These people have antibodies to Lyme but no symptoms. In people who do have symptoms show up over time, many of them improve with[cxviii] or without antibiotics.[cxix] [cxx] Over several years untreated Lyme arthritis patients get better.[cxxi] They can experience arthritic symptoms but those symptoms can fade.[cxxii] Following patients with symptoms treated briefly with antibiotics over a decade shows those symptoms can improve. After a decade, they did not have any more symptoms than the general population.[cxxiii]

In Norway, authorities estimate that over eight thousand people had Lyme rashes from tick bites every year. Of those, only three hundred people had more than a rash. Out of eight thousand, only eighty needed further care for Lyme symptoms. So while everyone in my endemic state knows someone with Chronic Lyme, the vast majority of us don't have it and won't get it.[cxxiv]

Interestingly, the same Norwegian study found that the

highest incidence of Lyme rashes were among older women.[cxxv] It is not a group I would commonly think of as being out in the woods as much as other groups. But they are a group more prone to autoimmune responses. If we make the comparison to rheumatoid arthritis, which shares genetic susceptibility with Chronic Lyme, the rate of higher infection among older women makes sense. Women get rheumatoid arthritis at twice the rate of men, and the incidence of rheumatoid arthritis rises for both sexes as we get older.[cxxvi]

Another study in Sweden found older women were fifty percent more likely to get rashes than younger women, and twice as likely to develop rashes as younger men. The Swedish study also estimated an overall Lyme rash rate at roughly five times as high as Norwegian authorities.[cxxvii]

In the Netherlands, authorities estimated that only one in sixty people bitten by a tick developed a rash.[cxxviii]

In the U.S., our rates of people reporting Lyme are lower than Norway, Sweden, or the Netherlands as a percentage of the population.[cxxix] We are not the most infectious place in the world, and most of the people in those more infectious places will never develop Chronic Lyme.

Yes, But...

None of this is helpful to any of us already experiencing ongoing symptoms from Chronic Lyme. At this point we need what ILADS doctors have to offer because we haven't gotten better on our own. Their expertise is in aggressively treating resistant Lyme and its co-infections. It's worthwhile to discuss our options with them and to consider a trial of treatment. We just want to keep in mind that we want them to make us feel better, not worse.

The way Lyme is being treated will be changing, because far more people are being diagnosed. Based on insurance numbers rather than the CDC, the rate of treating Chronic Lyme rose by fifty percent from 2006 to 2012.[cxxx] There isn't just more treatment, the treatment is more aggressive. A third of Chronic Lyme patients got two or more antibiotics in 2006, but that number had risen to half of all Chronic Lyme patients by 2012.

As the numbers of patients rise, more and more doctors will be better educated about Lyme. While ILADS likes to think of itself as being equal in size to the CDC, according to insurance reports less than five percent of doctors are prescribing antibiotics for more than twenty percent of all patients.[cxxxi] The diagnosed patients receiving extended antibiotic therapy were almost fifty percent more likely to have had a number of other health complaints in the previous three months.[cxxxii] So treating the Chronic Lyme may or may not resolve all their medical issues.

The number of patients and Lyme infections is likely to continue to rise. When we look at the history of one of Lyme's family of bacteria, syphilis, it can give us a view into the future of Lyme. Syphilis existed for many hundreds of years before it was recognized as a separate disease. Lyme was just recognized as a separate disease, although its history may go back five thousand years.[cxxxiii] Syphilis is still the third most common sexually transmitted disease, despite decades of trying to wipe it out. Lyme is not generally recognized as being sexually transmitted, but it very well may be.[cxxxiv] Syphilis is still susceptible to penicillin, but is showing resistance to the more advanced antibiotics.[cxxxv] Lyme has shown at least test-tube resistance to all of its common treatments. As antibiotic resistance spreads for syphilis and Lyme, plant-based novel antibiotics are the most likely route forward for both research and treatment.[cxxxvi]

Beyond ILADS

If we've been through the ILADS drug regimens and not improved it's time to take a bigger picture view of our condition. Can parts of the Chronic Lyme diagnosis be treated with another diagnosis? Muscle pain, arthritis, and fatigue may have other causes. If treatments for those causes are rapidly effective, none of us should begrudge anyone their journey to less pain regardless of the underlying diagnosis.

But the journey to health cannot rely on drugs. We need a method for correcting the body's immune response to Lyme. To shift it without suppressing it.

The question should shift from "how do we treat Lyme?" to "how do we treat an overactive immune system exposed to Lyme?" The goal isn't eradication of Lyme. It needs to be a life without any of the severe side effects of Lyme exposure.

Living with Lyme means living with the bacteria. It means understanding that exposure and re-exposure are near certainties. We need modification rather than attempted eradication. Efforts to eliminate Lyme without focusing on immune improvement are going to be fruitless and will weaken the patient more than the bacteria. We need to strengthen the patient while modifying the immune response.

10 Treating Lyme

I need to divide these treatment suggestions into four sections: life threatening, very painful/debilitating, mildly troubling, and no current symptoms.

No Current Symptoms

First, the easiest. No current symptoms. What should you do about your Chronic Lyme?

Absolutely nothing, because you don't have it. Yes, I'm sure your Lyme literate doctor wants you to do more. There are a million detox programs out there. But you do not have Chronic Lyme by any measure that makes any sense. Your antibody levels do not tell you if you have current Lyme or a past infection and there is no recognized test that will confirm you have Chronic Lyme. Most importantly, you don't have symptoms, which is the best possible outcome any ILADS doctor can promise you. No one on that side of the Lyme wars really believes that Chronic Lyme can be absolutely cured. So take your own life into your hands and walk away. If your aches and pains come back, OK, that brings you into the next group.

Mildly Troubling Symptoms

Rather than assume these are Lyme, treat them if you can as if they are the aches and pains of life. If they resolve with simple treatments or respond to other diagnoses, then treat them that way. Ordinarily, treating them as anything other than Chronic Lyme will involve less medication and be easier. Only if other treatments fail would you go into dramatic Lyme treatment.

Painful/Debilitating Symptoms: Herbs

We need lifelong treatments for those consistently troubled by chronic symptoms. These do not respond to other treatments and appear to most likely be Lyme. While antibiotics are exciting and enticing, the reality is that the cost and side effects of antibiotics make them a poor choice for lifelong treatment. We should reserve them for extreme situations (next section) when the side effect picture pales to the suffering caused by the Lyme itself. For low-grade Chronic Lyme care, the simplest treatment will be herbs. Eventually not herbs purchased, but herbs grown by patients or families themselves.

Herbalist Stephen Buhner is an expert in this area, and someone who has looked deeply at the Lyme situation. For those who want to know his basic protocol for Chronic Lyme, he posts it online.

(From other patients, I've heard that he's changed his protocol several times over the years. This is the most current protocol[cxxxvii] I was able to find.)

CORE PROTOCOL FOR LYME DISEASE

1. Japanese knotweed root (Polygonum cuspidatum) –up to three tbsps daily

2. Cat's claw (Uncaria tomentosa) –up to three tsps daily

3. Andrographis (Andrographis paniculata) –up to six capsules daily

Japanese Knotweed

If you want to follow Stephen Buhner's protocol and grow your own, Japanese Knotweed is an invasive plant that grows in Maine and elsewhere in the U.S. The Chinese herbal medicine form of the root may be effective against a variety of antibiotic-resistant bacteria.[cxxxviii] Evidently the young shoots can also be harvested and cooked like asparagus. It can also be prepared like rhubarb for an addition to jams and jellies.[cxxxix] The root contains the most resveratrol when harvested in October, but may vary in other compounds from Japanese or Chinese grown knotweed.[cxl] Still, it might be a viable commercial crop for resveratrol extraction as well as a homegrown treatment. Since it is invasive, take precautions about it escaping by potting it separately from the rest of the garden.

Cat's Claw

The other two ingredients in Buhner's basic herbs, cat's claw and andrographis, would need to be cultivated inside a greenhouse or purchased as powder in bulk. But interested readers should check with local farmers to see if a ready supply can't be gotten fresh.

Cat's claw is not terribly antibiotic, but it can be a good anti-inflammatory. Specifically for Chronic Lyme patients Cat's Claw can block an aspect of the immune cascade that seems to cause most, if not all, the worst symptoms.[cxli] Growing the plant is not usually done commercially, as the plant is normally harvested from the rainforest. But an indoor plant grown in partial shade should be a possibility in all climates.[cxlii] Unfortunately, the Peruvian government made exporting live cat's claw plants illegal, so finding even seeds may be difficult.[cxliii] A drug version, called CMED, uses a concentrated extract of cat's claw to prolong lymphocytes, the immune cells responsible for fighting viruses.[cxliv]

Andrographis

If you already know about Buhner's herbs, Buhner has written that andrographis is problematic because it only helps a little over half of those taking it. A few people get really severe allergic responses to the herb. But Buhner keeps it on the basics list because it is so effective when it does work.[cxlv] What we should know is that occasionally andrographis (and any herb) can cause anaphylactic shock level allergic reactions. A Thai study of andrographis found that immune compromised patients had a higher level of allergic response, and that the response could be delayed for some weeks. It was also a dose-dependent response, with higher doses of andrographis giving worse reactions.[cxlvi]

While I can't fault Buhner for his commitment to Lyme patients or his scholarship, the choices he has made for Lyme treatment can be difficult for people living in a world surrounded by Lyme. We need local Lyme solutions that can be locally grown, harvested, and used by those who need them.

Beyond Buhner

Moving beyond Buhner, a wide range of other herbs may be effective for Lyme treatment. Hundreds of plants have been tested for their effect on both ticks and on Lyme.

A recent review mentions many of these plants, including plants like teasel or oregano that have some popularity among the online Chronic Lyme crowd.

Twenty Herbal Compounds

Based on this one review, here are twenty compounds that could be used to block Chronic Lyme.[cxlvii]

1) Stevia rebaudiana- on spirochetes, round form, and biofilms.

2) Teasel (Dipsacus sylvestris)- on spirochetes

3) Grapefruit seed extract- on spirochetes, round form

4) Cat's Claw (Uncaria tomentosa) and Otoba parvifolia in combination- on spirochetes, round form, and biofilms

5) Wild cherry- on spirochetes, round form

6) Black walnut green hull- on spirochetes, round form, and biofilms

7) Apricot seed- on spirochetes, round form, and biofilms

8) Oregano- on spirochetes

9) Anise- on spirochetes, biofilms

10) Vitamin B complex- on spirochetes

11) Serrapeptase- on spirochetes, biofilms

12) Quercetin- on spirochetes, round form

13) E-viniferin- on spirochetes, round form

14) Resveratrol- on spirochetes, round form

15) Oleuropein- on spirochetes, round form

16) Amygdalin- on spirochetes, round form

17) Berberine sulphate- on spirochetes, round form

18) Apigenin- on spirochetes

19) Ellagic acid- on spirochetes

20) Malvidin- on spirochetes

Other compounds tried in this review did not show any effect on any of the Lyme forms. They include: white peony, olive leaf, sage, L-lysine, L-arginine, fulvic acid, and fucoidan.

Here we can easily fall into a classic ILADS doctor's trap of moving directly from the test tube trials to aggressive treatment. But with mild and moderate symptoms, the herbal side effects cannot outweigh the benefits received. We need herbs that help with Lyme, which have been widely used without severe side effects, and which are widely available without recourse to specialty herb supply stores. The last thing a patient needs is to find a helpful herb that is discontinued or perpetually out of stock.

Stevia

Going through the twenty compounds briefly, I will start with Stevia. The study on Stevia is startling, almost too good to be true. In a head-to-head trial, Stevia whole leaf extract outperformed other herbs. It also outperformed common antibiotics. Even when used in combination, doxycycline, cefoperazone, and daptomycin did not do as well as whole leaf Stevia in killing off all the forms of Lyme. The triple combination of antibiotics also triggered more biofilm growth, while Stevia decreased its growth.[cxlviii]

Let's be clear. Don't go out and buy the Stevia sweetener at the supermarket. Most of that has been purified to make it sweeter (like white sugar). What you want is a whole leaf extract. The products they used in the experiment were from Nutrametix, Now, Sweet Leaf, and Truvia. Only the Nutrametix whole leaf extract was at all effective. I'm not promoting them, because any whole leaf extract should be as effective (and I'm not a fan of their very expensive Chronic Lyme Protocols). It may also be that the research is not accurate or reproducible, so I would be cautious about depending on Stevia. But it certainly seems non-toxic and easier to swallow than many other herbs.

Teasel

Teasel is an herb promoted by herbalist Matthew Wood. To his credit, he recommends very small doses (up to nine drops). But Teasel is advertised as drawing out deep Lyme infection, and this review only found it effective on the most superficial form of the spirochete. Much of the herbal lore surrounding Teasel may come from Xu Duan (Dipsacus asperoides), the Chinese species. But in Matthew Wood's books he talks about the North American herb (Dipsacus sylvestris). Maine herbalist Deb Soule says the sylvestris works similarly, and one of her teachers was Matthew Wood.[cxlix] If that is the case, Xu Duan also shows significant progesterone activity, so that it could also alter patients hormonal levels if taken consistently.[cl]

Grapefruit Seed Extract

Grapefruit seed extract is a great antibiotic, antiviral, etc. for surface applications. Once it is absorbed by the body, there are several concerns. The first is whether the extract is authentic. Multiple case reports over the last several decades have found products claiming to contain grapefruit seed extract instead contain a synthetic antibiotic compound (benzethonium chloride).[cli] [clii] For surface cleaning this might be interchangeable. But internally the synthetic compound impacts the liver's functioning.[cliii]

Otoba

We've already talked about Cat's Claw from Buhner's

work. Adding Otoba parvifolia in combination is promoted by Dr. Marty Ross based on a Townsend article he read. But he also says that it outperforms antibiotics for him with his patients.[cliv] Very little research has been done on Otoba bark alone.

Wild Cherry Bark (Caution!)

Wild cherry bark (prunus serotina) contains amygdalin (number sixteen), the same compound found in apricot seeds (number seven). Enzymatic changes in the body can convert it to cyanide, making this a very toxic, but also a very powerful herb.[clv] Not one I would start with for mild to moderate Lyme symptoms.

Walnut Hull (Caution!)

Black walnut green hull (Juglans nigra) contains juglone, a compound that can also be gotten from an infusion (tea), but is absent from a decoction (extract). Juglone can sedate a variety of animals.[clvi] Dogs can be poisoned by it.[clvii] Some of the lore around the healing properties of black walnut may have come from Chinese medicine. But the Chinese species, Juglans regia, contains significantly different compounds.[clviii]

Apricot Seed (Caution!)

Apricot seed contains amygdalin (number sixteen). As an anti-tumor compound (Laetrile), amygdalin has not been shown to be effective. While any compound converting to cyanide in a test tube will kill Lyme spirochetes in the test tube, the estimated lethal dose of amygdalin for humans is around five grams.[clix]

Oregano

Oregano is a powerful antibacterial,[clx] antiviral,[clxi] etc. Fresh oregano is far superior, as stored oregano lost almost half its beneficial oils after three months.[clxii]

Anise

Anise is a surprising compound on this list, as I think of it as a mild member of the spice family. In testing for a range of spices as antibiotics, anise was outperformed by cumin, dill, and Turkish caraway.[clxiii] It was also less effective than black pepper or bay leaf, though it outperformed coriander.[clxiv] So anise's ability to destroy both the spirochete and round forms of Lyme raises great possibilities for the rest of the spice rack to be used in Chronic Lyme treatment.[clxv]

Vitamin B Complex

The vitamin B complex is not normally something I would consider an antibiotic. I know the synthetic form is a petrochemical creation, and certainly smells terrible. But I was unable to find even any online Lyme chatter of people using it to kill Lyme. It is often recommended as a supportive for Lyme recovery. If we move beyond the synthetic, it is likely that a nutritional yeast, Brewer's yeast, or even Saccharomyces boulardii[clxvi] might provide B complex for combating Lyme while also introducing competitive species. The S. boulardii could do that, interfering with Lyme's growth in the gut.

Serrapeptase

Serrapeptase is an enzyme that lowers body inflammation.[clxvii] It helps the body break down protein, and likely it breaks down the protein walls of the test tube Lyme. In patients, I would use it more for symptomatic relief of pain. It is classified as a drug in Japan and Europe.[clxviii]

Quercitin

Quercitin is widely available in many plants. It is commonly thought of as anti-inflammatory, but could also be anti-cancer and anti-viral.[clxix] Using Quercitin in combination with commonly used antibiotics can improve those antibiotics' effect.[clxx] The use of Quercitin itself would need to be in large amounts or with the extraction and concentration of its glycosides.[clxxi]

Resveratrol

E-viniferin is a Resveratrol dimer, a combination of two Resveratrol molecules. Resveratrol itself is of interest as an anti-cancer compound in large doses, though recent research has shown a benefit at much lower (dietary level) doses.[clxxii] While it is promoted strongly by multiple ILADS pioneers, recent research on Resveratrol shows that it might decrease the effects of other antibiotics and allow increased Lyme mutation.[clxxiii]

Oleuropein

Oleuropein is an extract of olive leaf or fruit. It is extracted from the green leaves or fruits of the plant, as its levels drop off when the fruit ripens. The extract is widely known as an anti-inflammatory, but also shows benefit against bacteria and viruses. The reason for its antibiotic effect is not entirely clear, but it contains compounds that may disrupt the building of cell walls.[clxxiv]

Amygdalin (Extreme Caution!)

Amygdalin is the cyanide compound found in wild cherry bark and apricot seeds. The release of this compound into the body varies by how much the gut bacteria breaks it down. So people on other antibiotics may be poisoned as they come off the antibiotics and their gut bacteria become more active.[clxxv]

Berberine

Berberine sulphate is a well-known herbal antibiotic that shows a broad range of effect on various bacterial species. It also may be effective on parasites.[clxxvi] The only downside is that it may be overharvested as it is commonly wild crafted from forests.

Apigenin

Apigenin is a plant flavone commonly thought of for its anti-cancer properties. It can be found in extracts of St. Johns Wort and chamomile, as well as foods like parsley and onions.[clxxvii] Its antibiotic effects may stem from its ability to encourage cell death.

Ellagic acid

Ellagic acid is a naturally occurring polyphenol that may, as an extract, block the clotting of blood.[clxxviii] Backing off the extract, a common source of the acid is the thornless blackberry (Rubus ulmifolius Schott), which may, in large quantities, block bacterial biofilm development.[clxxix] In lesser quantities, it can block bacterial growth without toxicity to the body's cells.

Malvidin

Malvidin is one of the pigments found in blueberries. It directly inhibits one of the inflammatory pathways generated by Lyme.[clxxx] It can also be found in wine and black carrots. The antibiotic effect may be from Malvidin blocking the communication between bacteria, which is a relatively new concept for antibiotics.[clxxxi]

Beyond Lists

We should not be limited in any way to this one list, nor fall into the trap of thinking of herbs as single entities. A single herb is a multitude of compounds and the combination of herbs provides us with greater benefit than the parts. We have also not looked at many of the more common compounds for Lyme, including green tea, garlic, or wormwood. I will address these later when I discuss my own treatment choices. But these are only a few of the many herbal options. One analysis within just the tradition of Ayurvedic medicine lists one hundred and seventy-five herbs that might be helpful with Lyme but which have not been tested against the spirochete, some of them familiar (ginger) and others far more exotic.[clxxxii]

Rosemary

One particular compound, rosmarinic acid, showed particular benefit (yes, we're talking kitchen spice rosemary, as in: parsley, sage, rosemary, and thyme). In ground testing to get rid of ticks, rosmarinic acid performed as well as an insecticide when sprayed on a lawn in a one part in ten solution.[clxxxiii] Orally, rosmarinic acid combined with vitamin D and vitamin C supported and increased the effect of doxycycline getting rid of Lyme.[clxxxiv] The combination of baicalein (from skullcap) and luteolin (from many plants) with either rosmarinic acid or iodine killed both spirochetes and round forms of Lyme while breaking down the biofilms that protect them.[clxxxv]

11 Treating Life-Threatening Lyme.

There are some people who need more than herbs. They need the strongest and fastest interventions possible to avoid dying of acute Lyme infection. These people are likely untreated Lyme patients who also have other diseases that have weakened their immune systems. In these cases we need to treat aggressively for Lyme, but limit treatments based on objective results. If nothing is improving, we should spend as little time with the patient "herxing" as possible before altering treatment. There are so many possible supportive treatments, it makes no sense to limit patients to any plan that isn't rapidly effective.

Once you've entered the life threatening level of Chronic Lyme, all of what has been said so far about "herxing" no longer applies. You need to do the most aggressive treatments regardless of "herxing" because your life hangs in the balance.

One hopeful aspect of severe Lyme is that the number of species of Lyme that can enter into the brain is far less diverse than those that can live elsewhere in the body. So if an aggressive treatment is effective, it is likely that the Lyme species within the brain will be wiped out.[clxxxvi]

Unfortunately, even the most aggressive common treatments may not be enough, particularly as Lyme antibiotic resistance spreads. So for those of you with loved ones in this situation, here is a list of twenty compounds that may help with systemic, life-threatening Lyme infection. They were selected from over four thousand compounds.

The researchers for this list found a hundred and fifty compounds that blocked over ninety percent of persisting, antibiotic-resistant Lyme. Of those, the FDA has approved over a hundred of these compounds for other uses. So the researchers picked the top twenty FDA approved compounds for use with very severe Lyme patients.

All of these top twenty compounds outperformed doxycycline for inhibiting Lyme growth (over 95%

reduction). And all have been FDA approved for other illnesses, so your doctors should be able to prescribe them in your state or country if they are available. For your doctor's sake, the following information comes from a Stanford University research team using a grant from the Bay Area Lyme Foundation (thanks to both of them!).

Here are the top twenty compounds to consider if facing life-threatening Lyme resistant to standard treatment.

1 Tetraethylthiuram disulfide

2 Doxorubicin hydrochloride

3 Josamycin

4 Cefotaxime acid

5 Cefazolin sodium

6 Epirubicin hydrochloride

7 Erythromycin ethylsuccinate

8 A-23187 calcimycin

9 Gramicidin

10 Cefdinir

11 Gambogic acid

12 Cephalothin sodium

13 Ceftazidime

14 Ticarcillin disodium

15 Valinomycin

16 Moxifloxacin hydrochloride

17 Linezolide

18 Idarubicin HCl

19 Tosufloxacin tosylate

20 Azlocillin sodium[clxxxvii]

Let's go through all twenty very briefly. Some of them are relatively common, while others are highly experimental.

The first compound, Tetraethylthiuram disulfide, is the drug Disulfuram. It is more commonly known as **Antabuse** and is used to treat alcoholism. The drug blocks the body's full breakdown of alcohol, leaving it as formaldehyde and poisoning a cheating alcoholic.

Doxorubicin hydrochloride, the second compound, was marketed as the anti-cancer drug Adriamycin PFS and is now a generic. Like most anti-cancer injectables, the side effect list is long.

The third compound, **Josamycin**, is a macrolide antibiotic available in many countries but may not be available in the U.S.

Number four, Cefotaxime acid or **Cefotamine**, is a third generation cephalosporin antibiotic. It works on a broad range of bacteria and is largely excreted in the urine.

Cefazolin sodium, number five, is a first generation cephalosporin antibiotic. It does not cross the blood brain barrier so would be less effective for neurological symptoms.

Our sixth compound, **Epirubicin** hydrochloride, is similar to number two, doxorubicin. It is another anti-cancer medication and may cause fewer side effects than doxorubicin.

Number seven, **Erythromycin** ethylsuccinate, or just erythromycin, is a well-known macrolide antibiotic.

A-23187 **calcimycin**, number eight, is a research antibiotic. It is described as "an ionophorous, polyether antibiotic from Streptomyces chartreusensis" by PubChem.

Our ninth compound, **Gramicidin**, is a heterogeneous mixture of six antibiotic peptides obtained from the soil bacterium Bacillus brevis. It is normally used topically, as its systemic effects can be severe.

Cefdinir, or **Omnicef**, is our tenth compound. It is a top selling third-generation cephalosporin antibiotic.

Number eleven, **Gambogic acid**, is a gum-resin from Southeast Asia. It is used as an anti-cancer drug. Gambogia also available as a homeopathic, where it is used to treat diarrhea.

Our twelfth compound, **Cephalothin** sodium (Cefalotin), is a beta-lactam, first-generation cephalosporin antibiotic. It may be marketed under a number of brand names.

Ceftazidime, or **Fortaz**, is our thirteenth compound. It is a third generation cephalosporin antibiotic administered intravenously or intramuscularly.

Our fourteenth compound, Ticarcillin disodium (**Ticar**) is a penicillin family antibiotic that is no longer manufactured alone. It may be available in combination with clavulanate potassium as Timentin.

Number fifteen, **Valinomycin**, is a potassium gradient antibiotic that is compared with number nine, Gramicidin, for overall effect. It has been used in experimental animal studies to reverse the lack of blood flow from stroke.

Moxifloxacin hydrochloride (**Avelox**), number sixteen, is a fluoroquinolone antibiotic, with the common side effects of that antibiotic class (tendon rupture, nerve effects).

Our seventeenth compound, Linezolide (**Zyvox**), is a Oxazolidinone antibiotic that interferes with a bacteria's ability to make proteins. It is used for the most resistant bacteria.

Idarubicin HCl, our eighteenth compound, is an anthracycline antineoplastic antibiotic (anti-cancer drug) that interferes with DNA synthesis. It penetrates cell membranes well and is used for leukemia and breast cancer.

Number nineteen, **Tosufloxacin** tosylate, is a fluoroquinolone antibiotic. It may not be available in the U.S., unlike number sixteen Moxifloxacin.

Our last compound, Azlocillin sodium (**Azlocillin**), is an extended range penicillin that may not be available in the U.S.

Other Studies

Other studies on new treatments for Lyme have focused purely on antibiotic options and found greater resistance from the Lyme bacteria than this study did.[clxxxviii] Branching out into other commonly used compounds (antimalarials, antifungals, etc.), many are more effective than the commonly used antibiotics while still leaving more than thirty percent of persistent Lyme bacteria alive.[clxxxix] Studies of extracts of Stevia (a plant sweetener) show more benefit than many of these prescription compounds.[cxc] Depending on the strain and history of the Lyme bacteria, different treatments may be more or less effective.

Focus On Persisters

But the current study of the top twenty listed above focused entirely on "persisters," antibiotic-resistant Lyme spirochetes. These are currently suspected to cause ongoing Lyme infection (unlike the other cell forms). Since it is likely that these "persister" spirochetes are the most troublesome for untreated Lyme patients with severe disease, this list of twenty was included..

Lesser Known "Cousin" Drugs

In the discussion section of this review, the researchers mentioned that both erythromycin and **kitasamycin** were very active compounds. Erythromycin was included on the list while kitasamycin, a similar macrolide antibiotic, was not. But since erythromycin is commonly used for Lyme perhaps the less well-known kitasamycin would be of more benefit to the same patients.

Of all the compounds listed, **Linezolide** (number seventeen) had a 98% reduction in Lyme bacteria persisters. It also has 100% bioavailability, making it one of the most effective compounds of the twenty.

Intracellular Lyme

For those concerned about the intracellular aspects of Lyme, **moxifloxacin** (number sixteen) has shown to be ten times more effective at destroying intracellular tuberculosis as other members of its antibiotic class. Another member of the same family, **tosufloxacin**, was almost as effective, blocking 97% of Lyme persister bacteria.

Beyond the Top Twenty

If none of the top twenty is sufficient to aid Chronic Lyme sufferers, **the study authors provided a listing of one hundred and twenty-eight additional compounds that block more than ninety-five percent of Lyme persister cells**. Readers can access the list (as S1) by following this endnote to the medline article.[cxci]

Beyond Search-And-Destroy

As we progress into the future of Lyme research, it may be that rotated dosing of Lyme with the right antibiotics will make a difference. But what is far more hopeful is research looking at the microbiome of the body and how it relates to Lyme. If we stop focusing only on the single spirochete bacteria and start looking at how it travels, feeds, and lives in our bodies, we may find new ways to compete with it.

In the old days, we thought of bacteria as invaders, and the body as defending itself against all the attacking hordes of bacteria. But over the last decade, we've started researching just how much we live with bacteria. Rather than a great wall, our bodies are porous. Bacteria live happily with us even inside the amniotic sac of an unborn child. (For more on this inner rainforest, see my book *Tending Your Internal Garden*.) So perhaps we do not need to eradicate or even concern ourselves as much with the Lyme spirochete. We need to instead engage in actively increasing the diversity of our inner ecosystems. We may find that one of the reasons that Lyme has become so virulent is because its natural competitors, non-disease causing spirochete bacteria,[cxcii] have been largely ignored and wiped out in our overly anxious modern hyper-hygienity. The very people who suffer the worst Chronic Lyme symptoms and who stay the cleanest may be the most desperately in need of a few more spirochetes, not less. A little more bacterial activity might down-regulate the overactive immune system.[cxciii] In the future, we may see probiotic (good bug) capsules containing harmless oral or skin spirochetes[cxciv] that can compete directly with Lyme for space in our bodies, forcing it into a minor role and allowing our immune systems to regulate, rather than overreact, to its presence.

Instead of the ongoing, fruitless debate over more or less antibiotics, doctors on both sides could come together to research and create novel protocols based on the experience of ILADS doctors over the last forty years. Treatments like cloning regulating immune cells and modifying the immune response with drug mimicry of down regulators are both feasible and being used for other immune diseases.[cxcv].

12 What I'm Going To Do

Prevention

Just say no. Just don't get bit. But imagine if you live in an endemic area like I do. Don't get bit is like saying don't get wet when you live in a lake. I'm going to get bit at some point.[cxcvi] My best preventative course is to disrupt the tick feeding cycle. If I focus my state government on deer and mouse feeding with anti-tick agents, I could possible drop my chances of getting bitten significantly (by 69%).[cxcvii]

If you believe the ILADers like Stephen Buhner, I'm eventually going to swap spit with someone who was bitten, or eat vegetables that might have encysted forms of Lyme on them from animal urine. In any case, I'm going to be exposed.

But maybe, you say, you could live in a permethrin-treated suit. Even then, suicidal tick nymphs will likely still bite me as they die.[cxcviii] Even though I should put down tick spray or rosemary oil on my yard to keep the ticks away, I love the fireflies too much to destroy their habitat just to give myself the illusion of safety.

I could move away down south where there aren't any Lyme ticks. But southern ticks spread STARI. It looks like Lyme, feels like Lyme, but the CDC is adamant that it's not Lyme.[cxcix] That's how silly the Lyme Wars have gotten.

The reality is that Lyme is less well recognized and treated elsewhere in the country. That and tornadoes keep me in Maine. Except that we had four tornadoes in Maine this past year. Oh well. (Falls on sword in despair).

One of the benefits of writing this book has been a decrease in my fear of getting bitten. By this point, I likely have been exposed and may not have noticed. If other biting insects are capable of spreading Lyme and its co-infections, then I've definitely been exposed. I recall huge "allergic" reactions to black fly and mosquito bites over the years. Now I suspect I was infected and fought off one or more of the co-infections or perhaps even Lyme itself. None of us should stop doing tick checks, but we should lose our panic if we find one. If we monitor the tick site, talk it over with our "Lyme friendly" doctor, and do what needs to be done, we should be fine. Don't assume the worst.

What we can do is constantly be treating ourselves with those "antibiotic" Lyme herbs that can be added to our cooking. I found the listing of anise as a Lyme killer extremely heartening, as it indicates that many of our common spices are likely to at least weaken any incoming Lyme spirochetes. So the best prevention may be constantly living a Lyme-resistant lifestyle. That means eating, drinking, sleeping and exercising to decrease inflammation and stress. The side effects of this kind of change are a drop in our risk of many other chronic diseases.

I'm going to cover the more conventional treatment options first, then discuss the herbs and other treatments as we reach the one year mark of treating Lyme. At that point most patients will have been through the best that even ILADS has to offer and be looking for other options.

Conventional Treatment: Getting Bitten

I'll get a script for doxycycline, but only take it if I'm sure it was a deer tick that had really gotten a piece of me. The script is just in case I start showing a rash, mounting a fever, or showing other symptoms. I know that partially treating Lyme is just going to screw up my ability to show up positive on the CDC lab tests while not giving me the protection I need.

Getting Symptoms

If/when I get bitten I'm going to get doxycycline to have on hand. A month's worth, to start with. And then I'm going to monitor how I feel. Even Stephen Buhner, the ILADS herbalist who wrote the book *Healing Lyme,* says 95% of people get better with antibiotics.

Knowing If I'm Better

Once I stop having symptoms I'm going to give it a few more days and stop taking antibiotics. If I don't feel worse, I'm going to stop worrying about Lyme. At this point I pretty much think any ILADS doctor who tells me I still have it when I don't have symptoms isn't someone I'd want to continue seeing.

Not Getting Better

Those that don't get better from antibiotics know they aren't better. Just like any patient that I've ever given anything to knows they're better or not. A patient who isn't better will say something like, "I do feel a little better." They're just being nice because they still feel terrible. In comparison, a truly better patient is either singing my praises or doesn't even mention the old aches because they've been gone for so long.

So if I'm not getting better from my Lyme, I'll know. My symptoms won't be completely gone. I'll still have a nagging illness that hasn't gone away. Being me, I'd likely ask for another month of antibiotics (as long as the side effects from the antibiotics aren't too nasty). Just another month to help my body beat the bug.

According to the CDC, I should never need a second month. But asking for a second month, particularly in a Lyme endemic area, shouldn't be that big a deal. Maybe I was re-exposed by another tick while recovering from the first one.

After Two Months of Antibiotics

After the second month, I'm likely to assume that antibiotics aren't going to work. I've read the ILADS literature that says I may need to take up to two years of the antibiotic to show a positive effect. But my reality check is that if it takes up to two years it might not be the antibiotics that eventually make the difference.

At this point, if not before, I'm going to look hard at the co-infections, particularly Babesia (Europeans would want to look at Bartonella, which is more common for them). Even without testing, I might request Babesia treatment.

In my mind Chronic Lyme symptoms could be either autoimmune at this point or an untreated co-infection. Since the other co-infections are somewhat treated by doxycycline, Babesia is my most likely culprit and first thing I'd treat. Now, part of me wants to treat for Babesia right off, but I will keep in mind that fifty-four Babesia cases were reported in Maine in 2015. Compare that to twelve hundred Lyme cases.[cc] We should treat for horse diseases like Lyme before we assume they are zebra diseases like Babesia.

Feeling Better On The Antibiotic, Worse Off It

What is also likely after the second month is that I might feel mostly better on the antibiotic and then get much worse when I'm off the antibiotic. In that case I might want to continue it because it lessens my symptoms. But not because I'm expecting it to do more than it did in the first week of treatment.

The improvement/worsening cycle of my symptoms is evidence that I have a low-grade ongoing infection and I need to rotate my antibiotics with additional support. It's the clearest indication that I need the help of an ILADS doctor who can oversee me with several combinations to really make an effort to overcome the ongoing infection.

By The Third Month

By the third month of treatment, I've likely left the CDC's model of Lyme and will need to find an ILADS doctor to prescribe me my antibiotic. While I would listen to his or her description of what is needed to eradicate Lyme (likely nine or more medications taken together), I'm not likely to try more than one at a time. I may not know what many ILADS doctors know about Lyme treatment, but I know my body doesn't like more than one medication at a time. So I'm more likely to try other things besides medications before I commit to years of aggressive, multi-drug treatment.

While ILADS talks about ending Lyme disease, a closer look at the ILADS literature makes this seem like an impossibility. It might be possible if you accepted the CDC's definition of Lyme infection as one kind of bacteria that can be killed easily by antibiotics. But the ILADS' definition of Lyme includes at least three kinds of each species of Lyme bacteria, including a wall-less form that hides within your own cells and a cyst form that's virtually impossible to kill. Both of these strange forms of Lyme bacteria make it extremely unlikely that a person with ILADS' defined Chronic Lyme will ever be truly free of Lyme.

The best we can hope for is to be healthy and feel well, virtually symptom-free despite having a few Lyme bacteria still in our bodies. Unless your ILADS doctor swears up and down that his or her treatment will absolutely wipe out all the Lyme in your body, the best you can hope for is to be symptom-free.

Getting Better Again

The second gruesome reality of the aggressive extended treatment and the perseverance of Lyme is the reality of re-exposure in any area where Lyme is endemic. As I showed in *Why Chronic Lyme Doesn't (And Does) Exist,* this area includes much of the world, certainly most of the U.S., Europe, and China. But it's also in areas like the Caribbean and even places like Egypt. So any Lyme treatment, no matter how effective, must take into account the very likely reality of re-exposure. Extremely intense treatments cannot be maintained year in and year out, and should be reserved only for the worst cases. They also should be done only until the cases have improved, weaning patients onto supportive care as soon as possible. Anyone treating Chronic Lyme as a single exposure capable of eradication is missing the forest for the trees. The goal has to be improvement and cure defined as living symptom-free rather than spirochete-free.

One Chronic Lyme patient I had in the past worked in a job where he was constantly re-exposed to deer tick bites. Whenever he was bitten again, he knew because every single previous bite on his body would flare up. He looked like he had chicken pox or the measles. But he was fortunate because a few days of doxycycline would resolve all his symptoms. Most of us don't have his exposure, but we can learn from his experience that even constant re-exposure is not a sentence for lifelong pain.

Active Spirochetes

But should we just allow the spirochetes to live within us? They don't, according to the CDC. ILADS can point to some biopsies that show very low numbers of the spirochetes continuing to exist in human tissue[cci] (the CDC has other biopsies that show they don't[ccii]). But the numbers of spirochetes found by ILADS doctors are not sufficient to cause the extreme symptoms that Chronic Lyme patients experience. So it is the body's reaction, not the presence of a few spirochetes, that causes most of the symptoms.

In an endemic world, think of Lyme in the same way you would a viral infection like herpes. In some studies, the herpes virus is shed in 98% of human tears.[cciii] That means it is everywhere. But relatively few people suffer from cold sores. And, while it does occur, convulsing and going into a coma from a herpes infection is extremely rare. (I once witnessed a case of herpes coma from Maine when I was in

Boston.) When severe events do happen it's likely the body is attacking the nerve tissue of the brain. The body wants to eradicate the herpes even when the herpes virus has intertwined itself into the core of the nerve tissue. So the only eradication possible is to eradicate the brain itself. We need to avoid this sort of "scorched earth" immune process with Lyme, keeping in mind that it is the patient's well-being and improved quality of life, not the delusion of our ability to eradicate every spirochete, that is the true goal of treatment. Symptom-free, not spirochete-free, is our goal.

After Six Months of Treatment

While I don't want to think about it, the reality is that if I came down with Chronic Lyme and didn't get better, I might still be sick after months. At that point I might be up for anything, trolling the internet and looking to start swallowing the salt or baking soda "cures" just in case they help. But because of this book, the first place I'd look is back at the co-infections, particularly Babesia or Anaplasma. If my symptoms are really bad, I might get another blood test even though they aren't conclusive. Rather than treating Chronic Lyme, I'd try another short course targeted just at getting rid of this particular co-infection. Realizing that antibiotics alone don't cure all the cases, I would focus my search on different plant compounds that might be effective.

After A Year: Autoimmune

As the months pass, the reality of my new chronically ill state would sink in. Instead of searching for a cure, I would realize that the likelihood is that I have an autoimmune response, not an ongoing infection. A number of drugs help significantly with autoimmune response.[cciv]

But that would not be the end of my journey, just the beginning. I know a fair amount about autoimmunity, but I don't need to know a ton to start making sure my life aligns with lowered inflammation. Knowing that sleep profoundly affects autoimmunity is a great start.[ccv] Behaviors like smoking will also profoundly increase my overall inflammation levels.[ccvi] I know that the inflammation levels of my gut, my microbiome, can impact how much pain and other symptoms I experience.[ccvii] With just this knowledge as a background, my journey to health involves bringing all of these areas into balance. Even if I don't attain complete symptom relief, my efforts may be rewarded by prolonging or even saving my life from other autoimmune issues like chronic heart disease.[ccviii]

For those of you who know about my colon cancer diagnosis (I'm in the second year of recovery), You won't be surprised that I'm already doing many of the things necessary to downplay autoimmunity and also prevent cancer recurrence.

Sleeping enough, exercising, and making less stressful lifestyle choices are all part of preventing and healing chronic illness of all kinds. We should not focus tightly on Chronic Lyme, because just dealing with Chronic Lyme over an extended period can lead to all the common side effects of having any chronic disease.

Anxiety, fatigue, rage, and depression are all part of the journey of chronic illness. They can be compounded with poverty from health care bills, the inability to work, and isolation from friends and social groups that do not recognize the validity of your diagnosis. Many of the symptoms of Chronic Lyme exemplify the common journey of the ill in our modern society.

In my own life, it turns out that being diagnosed with colon cancer provided that extra impetus I needed to stop my thirty-year "just this once" diet. We all know this diet, the one where you follow a good diet except for -just this once. The exceptions evidently resulted in my chronic allergies, two belt loops of belly fat, and chronic violent nightmares. Now that I skip "just this once" all of those have gone away.

The same diet I follow now is so full of anti-inflammatories that it puts any herbalist's protocol to shame. Forget teaspoons, I add tablespoons of good spices. I eat home cooked meals that contain the equivalent of a month's worth of those dry capsules many of you swallow every day with your fast food, drive through coffee. Please, none of you should think I'm judging. I'm constantly surprised every day that I haven't slid off the wagon yet.

It's good to feel good, but it's better to love feeling that way. My rule is that the day my body wants something junkie, it can have it. But so far, surprisingly, it hasn't.

I don't expect any of you to follow my diet, because I couldn't before my diagnosis. But if you've reached the end of your rope with chronic illness, it may be time to reach for something different.

Autoimmune Herbs

Unlike pharmaceutical drugs, herbs for autoimmunity may shift their character depending on the dose. A plant may be stimulating in a lower dose, but suppressing in a higher dose. The reality of herbs is that no one, not even the best herbal experts in the world, can tell you which of the three hundred plus compounds in a given pinch of herb will be the most reactive. It would be like predicting the quality of wine from a specific grapevine ten years in the future. There are too many variables. But that does not mean that we should not try different autoimmune herbs. Always taper up from the smallest dose, and remember that no one gets to tell you if something is a symptom of healing response or an herbal side effect. When it doubt, leave it out.

The herbs most interesting when looking at autoimmune moderation are those that both treat Lyme and also have immune moderating effects. These include berberine, apigenin, quercetin, Resveratrol, and E-viniferin. If they sound vaguely familiar, they are listed as Lyme spirochete killers and also make the short list for modifying immune responses. Unless you happen to like reading biochemistry books (and I suspect a little biochemistry knowledge is a modern day survival skill) there is an easier way to remember autoimmune moderating compounds that can be helpful in addition to the short list of herbs above. Did you get your "malvidin, delphinidin, cyanidin and petunidin aglycones" today? I bet you did. They are all the colored pigments found in blueberries. Nature's coloring agents, those bright oranges, reds, yellows and blues, are all immune moderating. So anything that naturally has those bright colors is likely to be good for you. It's as simple as going to the fresh section as you enter the supermarket and finding your color palette for the week.[ccix] Add to that list well know spices like pepper and rosemary, and most of us have something ready to hand in our kitchens that may both block Lyme growth and support our immune system into the bargain. [ccx]

We have also not looked at many of the more common compounds for Lyme, including garlic, green tea or wormwood.

Garlic inhibits the growth of babesia in mice.[ccxi] It blocks autoimmune brain damage at a human equivalent of five grams a day.[ccxii]

Green tea, at two grams a day, reduces autoimmune

response in Lupus patients.[ccxiii] At the human equivalent of one gram a day (for a 200 pound person), it blocks the growth the Babesia in cows and mice.[ccxiv]

Wormwood (Artemisia annua) is helpful in blocking a range of parasites including babesia.[ccxv] It is more effective than many antibiotics at killing off Lyme.[ccxvi] And an extract of wormwood may benefit autoimmune arthritis, so it may also help with Lyme autoimmunity.[ccxvii]

Many of the herbs helpful against Lyme (especially things like berberine and wormwood) can be very bitter. But adding whole leaf Stevia can certainly help with the taste. D-mannose, another sugar commonly used to prevent urinary tract infections, can also moderate the immune response and is being used in animal studies of diabetes and airway inflammation.[ccxviii] So you don't have to take the bitter herbs straight (unless you want to).

13 Update On Co-Infections

As I was getting this book ready for publication, Maine newspapers published terrifying stories about a massive increase in anaplasmosis and a doubling of babesia cases. While these are valid cases, they do not represent a major change in the infection rates, just a major change in diagnosing by local doctors. The rate of anaplasmosis nationwide has remained static, while Maine rates have climbed, stayed static and climbed again dramatically. The rates indicate the same underlying, ongoing infection rate, but with major changes in testing among urgent care and emergency room doctors.[ccxix] Maine reported 433 cases of anaplasmosis this year. Massachusetts, in comparison, reported 828 cases. Given the difference in population, are Mainers are five times more likely to get anaplasmosis from ticks that themselves have similar infection rates? It is far more likely that Mainers are five times more likely to be checked for anaplasmosis because Maine ER doctors are more aware of the problem and have made it a priority.[ccxx]

The rate of tick infection of Lyme, Anaplasma, and Babesia is very different. Five times as many ticks in Massachusetts have Lyme than have Anaplasma, and twice as many have Anaplasma as have Babesia.[ccxxi] Ticks from New York had similar rates of infection.[ccxxii] Older Maine tick surveys show a very gradual increase in cases of babesia, with a steady rate of Lyme infected ticks from 1995-2011.[ccxxiii] Surveys of ticks in Maine, Indiana, Wisconsin, and Pennsylvania found a higher rate of multiple infections within ticks, but they counted different species of the same bacteria as separate infections.[ccxxiv] The last survey of Maine published showed a sudden spike in anaplasmosis in 2008, but most testing did not check for erhlichiosis, which can give a false positive for anaplasmosis.[ccxxv]

The Maine rates of anaplasma exposure could be higher than the current human cases indicate. A Maine dog study found that 12% of dogs were positive for Lyme and 7% were positive for anaplasma. Vaccinating the dogs for Lyme dropped the infection rate from 15% to 10%, and using Lyme prevention sprays topically had no affect on infection rates.[ccxxvi]

According to the most recent CDC studies, the same treatment that will kill Lyme will also kill anaplasma. Mild babesia can be killed by azithromycin plus atovaquone.[ccxxvii]

For more herbal treatments for Anaplasma and Babesia, Stephen Buhner has listed off many herbs that could be helpful. In the medical journals we have almost no direct information about which herbs even kill anaplasma and babesia in a test tube. Rather than engage in a hunt-and-peck model of trying to find which herbs might work, I would begin with the ones that are 1) readily available, 2) have been shown through common use to be non-toxic long term, and 3) are helpful rather than making you feel worse.

14 Lyme Free Living

Until the time when medicine catches up to science in the study, diagnosis, and treatment of Lyme, there are a multitude of common changes we can make in our lives and lifestyles that down-regulate inflammation and encourage healing. All of these apply to Chronic Lyme as well as any of the host of other chronic autoimmune diseases.

In the Lyme tick itself, researchers have found that Lyme colonizes more when the immune system is more agitated. They can measure the success of Lyme in a tick based on how rapidly it can pass through the tissues.[ccxxviii] If the same model holds true for humans (a big leap), then an inflamed body may be exactly what Lyme prefers. The inflammation allows it to travel easily, moving from tissue to tissue at will.

Refocusing on Chronic Lyme as an autoimmune vs.

infectious illness opens the pathway to treating Chronic Lyme using immune regulation and modification strategies.

The core of any lifestyle program must be the lifestyle. So sleeping, eating, playing and socializing are not optional if you get your daily supplements. Skip the pills and live better.

Generally, people do better sleeping in hour-and-a-half segments. Four or five of these every night (six to seven and a half hours) is the most healthy.

Eating like a person in the Mediterranean is healthier. But this includes preparing food, taking the time to eat it, and socializing during eating. Wolfing down a frozen Mediterranean dinner for one while watching the news misses the point.

A diet rich in natural colors, full of fruits and vegetables, provides significant quantities of Lyme fighting material relatively painlessly.

A huge part of the Mediterranean diet is the addition of spices. Recalling the chapters on Lyme fighting herbs, these should be part of the daily palette for food. Anyone who decides to swallow oregano as a pill without using oregano in their cooking is only gaining the biochemistry of the herb while missing the savor.

Speaking of savor, walking is the stuff of life. The jumping programs and high-tech fifteen second workouts fail to activate the healing response in the human body. Walking for an hour a day sets up inflammation and resolution, boosting the best blend of immune modulation. Nothing faster or more intense outperforms the gentle rhythms of the body.

Engaging with others while walking and eating are critical to the healing of the body. We are a lonely people, seeking community through the ether. But we should remember that even premature infants know the healing power of touch. It's not optional to be part of your community, it's essential to understand the social nature of who we are and how we relate on a personal level. Until the time comes that a thumbs up literally feels like a hug, spend as much time with real people as you do with virtual ones.

Patients with Chronic Lyme, and all of us who live in an endemic world, can feel hopeful that the combination of our natural innate immune response and medical ingenuity can still bring us to a healthy, symptom-free life.

ABOUT THE AUTHOR

Dr. Christopher Maloney, N.D., lives in Lyme endemic Maine with a dog who has Lyme but doesn't show symptoms (yet). He (the doctor, not the dog) looks forward to long winters when the ticks are frozen. In his practice, Dr. Maloney works with Chronic Lyme patients who have been through Chronic Lyme treatments without great success. Together they try to put together a life plan for health.

I hope and pray that something in this book will be helpful to you. If even one of my readers benefits, then my work will be rewarded.

Please review my work on your favorite reading list. You are the most trustworthy and powerful source of help for your community. Let them know what helps you.

Thank you.

---

[i] http://www.nejm.org/doi/full/10.1056/NEJMe1502350#t=article

[ii] https://www.ncbi.nlm.nih.gov/pubmed/21196901

[iii] https://www.ncbi.nlm.nih.gov/pubmed/17578771

[iv] https://www.ncbi.nlm.nih.gov/pubmed/17578772

[v] http://www.nejm.org/doi/full/10.1056/NEJMe1502350#t=article

[vi] https://www.niaid.nih.gov/diseases-conditions/lyme-disease

[vii] http://www.tandfonline.com/doi/full/10.1586/14787210.2014.940900

[viii] https://www.ncbi.nlm.nih.gov/pubmed/28681315

[ix] https://www.ncbi.nlm.nih.gov/pubmed/8556471

[x] https://www.ncbi.nlm.nih.gov/pubmed/27612442

[xi] https://www.ncbi.nlm.nih.gov/pubmed/11693973

[xii] https://www.ncbi.nlm.nih.gov/pubmed/23190290

[xiii] https://www.ncbi.nlm.nih.gov/pubmed/28365751

[xiv] https://www.ncbi.nlm.nih.gov/pubmed/18452807

[xv] https://www.ncbi.nlm.nih.gov/pubmed/3885366

[xvi]http://www.ct.gov/dph/lib/dph/infectious_diseases/lyme/1976_circular_letter.pdf

[xvii] https://www.cdc.gov/lyme/treatment/prolonged/index.html

[xviii] https://www.ncbi.nlm.nih.gov/pmc/articles/PMC4075423/

[xix] ILADS-patient factsheet, 2017.http://ilads.org/lyme/getlymesmart.pdf

[xx] https://www.ncbi.nlm.nih.gov/pmc/articles/PMC4480264/

[xxi] https://www.ncbi.nlm.nih.gov/pubmed/25182244

[xxii] https://www.ncbi.nlm.nih.gov/pmc/articles/PMC86513/

[xxiii] http://www.nejm.org/doi/10.1056/NEJM200107123450202

[xxiv] https://www.ncbi.nlm.nih.gov/pubmed/8877079

[xxv] https://www.ncbi.nlm.nih.gov/pubmed/28365751

[xxvi] https://www.ncbi.nlm.nih.gov/pubmed/28148307

[xxvii] https://www.ncbi.nlm.nih.gov/pubmed/20382722

[xxviii] https://www.ncbi.nlm.nih.gov/pubmed/27931077

[xxix] https://www.ncbi.nlm.nih.gov/pubmed/27686962

[xxx] https://www.ncbi.nlm.nih.gov/pubmed/26607686

[xxxi] https://www.ncbi.nlm.nih.gov/pubmed/27013465

[xxxii] https://www.ncbi.nlm.nih.gov/pubmed/26459093

[xxxiii] https://www.ncbi.nlm.nih.gov/pubmed/16530006

[xxxiv] https://www.ncbi.nlm.nih.gov/pmc/articles/PMC4196523/

[xxxv] https://www.ncbi.nlm.nih.gov/pubmed/9455520

[xxxvi] https://www.ncbi.nlm.nih.gov/pmc/articles/PMC4252587/

[xxxvii] https://www.ncbi.nlm.nih.gov/pubmed/3591095

[xxxviii] https://www.ncbi.nlm.nih.gov/pubmed/2065539

[xxxix] https://www.ncbi.nlm.nih.gov/pubmed/27408074

[xl] https://www.ncbi.nlm.nih.gov/pubmed/25239124

[xli] https://data.mainepublichealth.gov/tracking/lyme-2016update

[xlii] https://www.ncbi.nlm.nih.gov/pubmed/2063950

[xliii] https://www.ncbi.nlm.nih.gov/pubmed/8905312

[xliv] https://www.ncbi.nlm.nih.gov/pubmed/1941949

[xlv] https://www.ncbi.nlm.nih.gov/pubmed/10703202

[xlvi] http://www.nejm.org/doi/full/10.1056/NEJM199006143222415

[xlvii] https://www.ncbi.nlm.nih.gov/pubmed/3170711

[xlviii] https://www.ncbi.nlm.nih.gov/pubmed/18274258

[xlix] https://www.ncbi.nlm.nih.gov/pubmed/28690828.3

[l] https://www.ncbi.nlm.nih.gov/pubmed/20925520

[li] https://www.ncbi.nlm.nih.gov/pubmed/7648832

[lii] https://www.ncbi.nlm.nih.gov/pubmed/17225014

[liii] https://www.cdc.gov/media/releases/2016/p0208-lyme-disease.html

[liv] https://www.ncbi.nlm.nih.gov/pmc/articles/PMC3565243/#R272

[lv] https://www.ncbi.nlm.nih.gov/pubmed/19017912

[lvi] https://www.ncbi.nlm.nih.gov/pubmed/17043300

[lvii] https://www.ncbi.nlm.nih.gov/pubmed/28748396

[lviii] https://www.fda.gov/ohrms/dockets/ac/01/briefing/3680b2_03.pdf

[lix] https://www.ncbi.nlm.nih.gov/pubmed/21217173

[lx] https://www.ncbi.nlm.nih.gov/pubmed/9685265

[lxi] https://www.ncbi.nlm.nih.gov/pubmed/28141584

[lxii] https://www.ncbi.nlm.nih.gov/pmc/articles/PMC3216572/

[lxiii] https://www.ncbi.nlm.nih.gov/pmc/articles/PMC2647156/

[lxiv] https://www.ncbi.nlm.nih.gov/pmc/articles/PMC4231398/

[lxv] https://www.hindawi.com/journals/ad/2012/539282/

[lxvi] https://www.ncbi.nlm.nih.gov/pmc/articles/PMC1005560/

[lxvii] https://www.ncbi.nlm.nih.gov/pmc/articles/PMC3106239/

[lxviii] https://www.ncbi.nlm.nih.gov/pubmed/3668982

[lxix] https://www.ncbi.nlm.nih.gov/pubmed/109097

[lxx] https://www.ncbi.nlm.nih.gov/pubmed/503166

[lxxi] https://www.ncbi.nlm.nih.gov/pmc/articles/PMC2430045/

[lxxii] https://www.ncbi.nlm.nih.gov/pmc/articles/PMC4657537/

[lxxiii] https://www.ncbi.nlm.nih.gov/pubmed/28617768

[lxxiv] https://www.ncbi.nlm.nih.gov/pubmed/28077740

[lxxv] https://www.ncbi.nlm.nih.gov/pubmed/16288069

[lxxvi] https://www.ncbi.nlm.nih.gov/pubmed/28077740

[lxxvii] https://www.ncbi.nlm.nih.gov/pubmed/20091554

[lxxviii] https://www.wired.com/2009/08/ff-placebo-effect/

[lxxix] https://www.ncbi.nlm.nih.gov/pubmed/11049799

[lxxx] https://www.ncbi.nlm.nih.gov/pubmed/6752295

[lxxxi] https://www.ncbi.nlm.nih.gov/pubmed/3723728

[lxxxii] https://www.ncbi.nlm.nih.gov/pubmed/9511083

[lxxxiii] https://www.ncbi.nlm.nih.gov/pubmed/28077740

[lxxxiv] https://www.ncbi.nlm.nih.gov/pmc/articles/PMC3608636/

[lxxxv] https://www.ncbi.nlm.nih.gov/pubmed/16455348

[lxxxvi] https://www.ncbi.nlm.nih.gov/pubmed/8663853

[lxxxvii] https://www.ncbi.nlm.nih.gov/pubmed/28711878

[lxxxviii] https://www.ncbi.nlm.nih.gov/pubmed/28175297

[lxxxix] https://www.ncbi.nlm.nih.gov/pubmed/25922085

[xc] https://www.ncbi.nlm.nih.gov/pubmed/3591091

[xci] https://www.ncbi.nlm.nih.gov/pubmed/6842024

[xcii] https://www.ncbi.nlm.nih.gov/pubmed/14935211

[xciii] https://www.ncbi.nlm.nih.gov/pubmed/6752295

[xciv] https://www.ncbi.nlm.nih.gov/pubmed/9610974

[xcv] https://www.ncbi.nlm.nih.gov/pubmed/12893393

[xcvi] https://www.ncbi.nlm.nih.gov/pmc/articles/PMC4490322/

[xcvii] https://www.ncbi.nlm.nih.gov/pubmed/1260219

[xcviii] https://articles.mercola.com/sites/articles/archive/2009/03/14/clearing-up-confusion-on-vitamin-d--why-i-dont-recommend-the-marshall-protocol.aspx

[xcix] https://www.ncbi.nlm.nih.gov/pmc/articles/PMC2912737/

[c] https://www.ncbi.nlm.nih.gov/pmc/articles/PMC473601/?page=1

[ci] https://www.ncbi.nlm.nih.gov/pubmed/12576359

[cii] https://www.ncbi.nlm.nih.gov/pubmed/28408469

[ciii] https://www.ncbi.nlm.nih.gov/pmc/articles/PMC5052740/#RSTB20150494C28

[civ] https://www.ncbi.nlm.nih.gov/pmc/articles/PMC172922/pdf/100320.pdf

[cv] https://www.ncbi.nlm.nih.gov/pubmed/15651712

[cvi] https://www.ncbi.nlm.nih.gov/pubmed/24336823/

[cvii] https://www.ncbi.nlm.nih.gov/pubmed/8565717

[cviii] https://rawlsmd.com/

[cix] https://joettecalabrese.com/blog/protocol-lyme-disease-using-homeopathy/

[cx] http://ndnr.com/pain-medicine/chronic-tick-borne-infections-relief-using-bee-venom-treatment/

[cxi] https://www.ncbi.nlm.nih.gov/pubmed/3763815

[cxii] https://www.ncbi.nlm.nih.gov/pubmed/7479280

[cxiii] https://www.cdc.gov/parasites/babesiosis/health_professionals/index.html

[cxiv] https://www.ncbi.nlm.nih.gov/pubmed/8637139

[cxv] http://www.aafp.org/afp/2001/0515/p1969.html

[cxvi] https://www.ncbi.nlm.nih.gov/pmc/articles/PMC3998201/

[cxvii] https://academic.oup.com/cid/article/32/8/1117/477798/Severe-Babesiosis-in-Long-Island-Review-of-34

[cxviii] https://www.ncbi.nlm.nih.gov/pubmed/28277054

[cxix] https://www.ncbi.nlm.nih.gov/pubmed/26028977

[cxx] https://www.ncbi.nlm.nih.gov/pubmed/3662285

[cxxi] http://onlinelibrary.wiley.com/doi/10.1002/art.22131/full

[cxxii] https://www.ncbi.nlm.nih.gov/pmc/articles/PMC2907555/

[cxxiii] https://www.ncbi.nlm.nih.gov/pubmed/25888674

[cxxiv] https://www.ncbi.nlm.nih.gov/pubmed/27475874

[cxxv] https://www.ncbi.nlm.nih.gov/pubmed/27475874

[cxxvi] https://rheumatoidarthritis.net/what-is-ra/ra-statistics/

[cxxvii] https://www.ncbi.nlm.nih.gov/pubmed/17417955

[cxxviii] https://www.ncbi.nlm.nih.gov/pubmed/25448421

[cxxix] https://www.ncbi.nlm.nih.gov/pubmed/26291194

[cxxx] https://www.ncbi.nlm.nih.gov/pubmed/26393537

[cxxxi] https://www.ncbi.nlm.nih.gov/pubmed/26223992

[cxxxii] https://www.ncbi.nlm.nih.gov/pubmed/27855040

[cxxxiii] http://news.nationalgeographic.com/news/2013/10/131016-otzi-ice-man-mummy-five-facts/

[cxxxiv] https://www.ncbi.nlm.nih.gov/pubmed/28690828.3

[cxxxv] https://www.ncbi.nlm.nih.gov/pubmed/19805553

[cxxxvi] https://www.ncbi.nlm.nih.gov/pubmed/25683888

[cxxxvii] http://buhnerhealinglyme.com/the-protocols/

[cxxxviii] https://www.ncbi.nlm.nih.gov/pubmed/26087259

[cxxxix] http://mainekitchen.bangordailynews.com/2014/05/06/japanese-knotweed-invasive-and-tasty/

[cxl] https://www.ncbi.nlm.nih.gov/pubmed/23742076

[cxli] https://www.ncbi.nlm.nih.gov/pubmed/19995599

[cxlii] https://www.hort.purdue.edu/newcrop/CropFactSheets/catsclaw.html

[cxliii] https://www.richters.com/show.cgi?page=QandA/Growing/19991106-1.html

[cxliv] https://www.ncbi.nlm.nih.gov/pubmed/12622460

[cxlv] http://buhnerhealinglyme.com/herbs/why-dont-you-recommend-andrographis-anymore/

[cxlvi] https://www.ncbi.nlm.nih.gov/pmc/articles/PMC4364323/

[cxlvii] https://www.ncbi.nlm.nih.gov/pmc/articles/PMC4971593/#bibr45-2049936116655502

[cxlviii] https://www.ncbi.nlm.nih.gov/pmc/articles/PMC4681354/

[cxlix] https://www.youtube.com/watch?v=3-aEQYk3hs0

[cl] https://www.ncbi.nlm.nih.gov/pubmed/24845509

[cli] https://www.ncbi.nlm.nih.gov/pubmed/11453769

[clii] https://www.ncbi.nlm.nih.gov/pubmed/18344660

[cliii] https://www.ncbi.nlm.nih.gov/pubmed/17468864

[cliv] http://www.treatlyme.net/treat-lyme-book/otoba-bark-extract-and-cats-claw-tinctures/

[clv] http://www.planetherbs.com/michaels-blog/wild-cherry-one-of-the-great-north-american-herbs.html

[clvi]https://www.ncbi.nlm.nih.gov/pubmed/14006337

[clvii] https://www.ncbi.nlm.nih.gov/pubmed/26720086

[clviii]https://www.ncbi.nlm.nih.gov/pubmed/24354208

[clix] http://www.cancerjournal.net/article.asp?issn=0973-1482;year=2014;volume=10;issue=5;spage=3;epage=7;aulast=Song

[clx] https://www.ncbi.nlm.nih.gov/pubmed/19783523

[clxi] https://www.ncbi.nlm.nih.gov/pubmed/24779581

[clxii] https://www.ncbi.nlm.nih.gov/pubmed/25177730

[clxiii] https://www.ncbi.nlm.nih.gov/pubmed/12410554

[clxiv] https://www.ncbi.nlm.nih.gov/pubmed/16935829

[clxv] https://www.ncbi.nlm.nih.gov/pubmed/26991289

[clxvi] https://www.ncbi.nlm.nih.gov/pubmed/2494098

[clxvii] https://www.ncbi.nlm.nih.gov/pubmed/6366808

[clxviii] https://www.ncbi.nlm.nih.gov/pubmed/23380245

[clxix] https://www.ncbi.nlm.nih.gov/pubmed/26999194

[clxx] https://www.ncbi.nlm.nih.gov/pubmed/25879586

[clxxi]https://www.ncbi.nlm.nih.gov/pubmed/24320230

[clxxii] https://www.ncbi.nlm.nih.gov/pmc/articles/PMC4827609/

[clxxiii] https://www.ncbi.nlm.nih.gov/pmc/articles/PMC4821490/

[clxxiv] https://www.ncbi.nlm.nih.gov/pmc/articles/PMC3002804/

[clxxv] https://www.ncbi.nlm.nih.gov/pmc/articles/PMC1272529/

[clxxvi] https://www.ncbi.nlm.nih.gov/pmc/articles/PMC4289877/

[clxxvii] https://www.ncbi.nlm.nih.gov/pmc/articles/PMC2874462/

[clxxviii] https://www.ncbi.nlm.nih.gov/pubmed/25037345

[clxxix] https://www.ncbi.nlm.nih.gov/pubmed/22242149

[clxxx] https://www.ncbi.nlm.nih.gov/pubmed/24333549

[clxxxi]http://www.sciencedirect.com/science/article/pii/S088240101500011X?via%3Dihub

[clxxxii] https://www.ncbi.nlm.nih.gov/pmc/articles/PMC3170500/

[clxxxiii] https://www.ncbi.nlm.nih.gov/pubmed/20695287

[clxxxiv] https://www.ncbi.nlm.nih.gov/pubmed/27570483

[clxxxv] https://www.ncbi.nlm.nih.gov/pubmed/28644529

[clxxxvi] https://www.ncbi.nlm.nih.gov/pubmed/21829670

[clxxxvii] https://www.ncbi.nlm.nih.gov/pmc/articles/PMC4827596/

[clxxxviii] https://www.ncbi.nlm.nih.gov/pmc/articles/PMC4126181/

[clxxxix] https://www.ncbi.nlm.nih.gov/pmc/articles/PMC4790293/

[cxc] https://www.ncbi.nlm.nih.gov/pmc/articles/PMC4681354/

[cxci] https://www.ncbi.nlm.nih.gov/pmc/articles/PMC4827596/table/ts1-dddt-

10-1307/

[cxcii] https://www.ncbi.nlm.nih.gov/pubmed/1238163

[cxciii] https://www.ncbi.nlm.nih.gov/pubmed/27170508

[cxciv] http://www.blackwellreference.com/public/tocnode?id=g9781405161695_chunk_g978140516169530_ss728

[cxcv] https://www.ncbi.nlm.nih.gov/pubmed/24924121

[cxcvi] https://www.ncbi.nlm.nih.gov/pubmed/11444404

[cxcvii] https://www.ncbi.nlm.nih.gov/pubmed/16524769

[cxcviii] https://www.ncbi.nlm.nih.gov/pubmed/15061284

[cxcix] https://www.ncbi.nlm.nih.gov/pubmed/18452807

[cc] http://www.maine.gov/dhhs/mecdc/infectious-disease/epi/vector-borne/lyme/index.shtml

[cci] https://www.ncbi.nlm.nih.gov/pubmed/1980573

[ccii] https://www.ncbi.nlm.nih.gov/pubmed/8506882

[cciii] https://www.ncbi.nlm.nih.gov/pmc/articles/PMC1200985/

[cciv] https://www.ncbi.nlm.nih.gov/pmc/articles/PMC4548092/

[ccv] https://www.ncbi.nlm.nih.gov/pubmed/26402614

[ccvi] https://www.ncbi.nlm.nih.gov/pubmed/18037930

[ccvii] https://www.ncbi.nlm.nih.gov/pubmed/26953630

[ccviii] https://www.ncbi.nlm.nih.gov/pubmed/18991025

[ccix] https://www.ncbi.nlm.nih.gov/pmc/articles/PMC5537178/

[ccx] https://www.ncbi.nlm.nih.gov/pmc/articles/PMC4548092/

[ccxi] https://www.ncbi.nlm.nih.gov/pubmed/24173810

[ccxii] https://www.ncbi.nlm.nih.gov/pubmed/28939293

[ccxiii] https://www.ncbi.nlm.nih.gov/pubmed/28585735

[ccxiv] https://www.ncbi.nlm.nih.gov/pubmed/20025823

[ccxv] https://www.ncbi.nlm.nih.gov/pubmed/27867026

[ccxvi] https://www.ncbi.nlm.nih.gov/pmc/articles/PMC4790293/

[ccxvii] https://www.ncbi.nlm.nih.gov/pubmed/27411673

[ccxviii] https://www.ncbi.nlm.nih.gov/pubmed/28759052

[ccxix] http://maine.gov/dhhs/mecdc/infectious-disease/epi/vector-borne/anaplasmosis/documents/Anaplasma-2015.pdf

[ccxx] http://www.pressherald.com/2017/11/13/anaplasmosis-cases-surging-in-maine/

[ccxxi] https://www.ncbi.nlm.nih.gov/pubmed/27248292

[ccxxii] https://www.ncbi.nlm.nih.gov/pubmed/24605473

[ccxxiii] https://www.ncbi.nlm.nih.gov/pmc/articles/PMC4193268/

[ccxxiv] https://www.ncbi.nlm.nih.gov/pubmed/18402145

[ccxxv] https://www.ncbi.nlm.nih.gov/pubmed/19779398

[ccxxvi] https://www.ncbi.nlm.nih.gov/pmc/articles/PMC3321752/

[ccxxvii] https://www.ncbi.nlm.nih.gov/pubmed/27115378

[ccxxviii] http://www.yalescientific.org/2014/04/modulated-colonization-of-the-bacteria-that-cause-lyme-disease/

Made in the USA
Middletown, DE
08 September 2024

60641540R00096